MOLLY FOX'S YOGA

WEIGHT LOSS PROGRAM

The Stress-Free Way to Get the Body You Love

By Molly Fox and Jonny Bowden, M.A., C.N., C.N.S.

A
Adams Media
Avon, Massachusetts

Dedications

To my mom and dad. —Molly

For my mother, with eternal gratitude for
all your unconditional love and support. —Jonny

Published by
Adams Media, an F+W Publications Company
57 Littlefield Street, Avon, MA 02322. U.S.A.
www.adamsmedia.com

ISBN: 1-59337-010-5

Printed in The United States of America.

J   I   H   G   F   E   D   C   B   A

Library of Congress Cataloging-in-Publication Data
Fox, Molly.
[Yoga weight loss program]
Molly Fox's yoga weight loss program / Molly Fox and Jonny Bowden.
p.   cm.
ISBN 1-59337-010-5
1. Weight loss. 2. Yoga. 3. Reducing exercises.
I. Title: Yoga weight loss program.
II. Bowden, Jonny. III. Title.
RM222.2.F679 2004
613.2'5--dc22

2003022377

This publication is designed to provide accurate and authoritative information with regard to the subject matter covered. It is sold with the understanding that the publisher is not engaged in rendering legal, accounting, or other professional advice. If legal advice or other expert assistance is required, the services of a competent professional person should be sought.
—From a *Declaration of Principles* jointly adopted by a Committee of the American Bar Association and a Committee of Publishers and Associations

Many of the designations used by manufacturers and sellers to distinguish their products are claimed as trademarks. Where those designations appear in this book and Adams Media was aware of a trademark claim, the designations have been printed with initial capital letters.

Molly Fox's Yoga Weight Loss Program is intended as a reference volume only, not as a medical manual. In light of the complex, individual, and specific nature of health problems, this book is not intended to replace professional medical advice. The ideas, procedures, and suggestions in this book are intended to supplement, not replace, the advice of a trained medical professional. Consult your physician before adopting the suggestions in this book, as well as about any condition that may require diagnosis or medical attention. The authors and publisher disclaim any liability arising directly or indirectly from the use of this book.

©Interior Photography by Gina Fong
This book is available at quantity discounts for bulk purchases.
For information, call 1-800-872-5627.

Contents

Acknowledgments

This book could not have been made without the enormous contributions of so many people. This includes all the people who have served as my teachers, way before this process and of course during the process of writing this book.

Thanks to . . .

First and foremost John Friend, the creator of Anusara Yoga. Thank you for teaching me how to hold the practice of teaching yoga in my heart.

Special thanks to Rebecca Thomas, Tevis Trower, Jenny Otto, Jackie Prete, Jennifer Brilliant, Joan Arnold, Diana Rilov, Kerry Silverstone, Caroline Kohles (all the NYC NIA folks), and Michael Port, who create a soft place for me to fall and teach me about friendship.

A special shout out to all of my students. You guys, I love you, and you have taught me so much about honor and commitment. Especially those who followed me from Molly Fox Studios to Equinox Fitness Clubs and put up with all of my learning curves.

Judy Talesnick, Dave Buck, Cynthia Merchant, Michael Ray, Siddha Yoga, Lorna Catford, Patricia Simko, and the Universal Presence.

My two sisters, Julie Daley and Katie Peuvrelle, who bared all and gave so much of their time to be in the photographs inside this book. Don't they look awesome?

A special thanks to Katie Peuvrelle, who as an amazing hypnotherapist and sport and performance coach contributed the chapter on self-hypnosis.

My daughter Liza, who supports me like crazy. My whole extended family, Mom, Dad, and the bunch for being the greatest family in the world and my two furry buddies Max and Grace Kali for teaching me about the natural world and reminding me I am an animal and not an iMac.

Gina Fong and Gina Fong Photography for all the stunning pictures. You are the best girlfriend.

And of course, Linda Konner, Nancy Stedman, Gary Krebs, Courtney Nolan, and all the folks at Adams Media and the phenomenal Jonny Bowden who makes collaborative writing a juicy, fun e-ride type of party. Thanks for sharing the birthing process.

Who We Are

The things that matter most must never be at the mercy of those which matter least.

—Johann Wolfgang von Goethe (1749–1832)

Introducing Molly Fox (by Jonny Bowden)

I first met Molly 25 years ago when we were both students at the Actors Institute in New York. At the time, she was a dancer and I was a pianist. The Actors Institute was a very special kind of school; started by some graduates of what is now the Landmark Forum, its mission was to help people in the arts become more fully self-expressed. It was less an acting school than a place where you could learn to break through barriers—usually of your own making—that kept you from being as big in the world as you could be and from making as bold a statement (on stage and off) and as big a contribution as you were capable of. At one point the instructor had us go around the room and state our biggest dream. When it came to Molly, she stood up and said, just as big and bold and proud as she could be, "I want to teach aerobics in New York City and be successful at it!"

Twenty-five years ago, achieving this goal was no small task for a young girl new to New York. Molly had a love for movement and fitness, but no teaching experience in the cutthroat Big City—plus there was competition from heavyweight established aerobic "stars."

Six months later, the Molly Fox Studio was born out of a rented dance space within the building owned by the Actors Institute. On a good day, Molly would teach one class a day there and consider herself lucky if there were 10 people in attendance. But not for long. Slowly but surely I watched her class build until eventually you could hardly get into the lobby area, as students in spandex and leg warmers crowded the hallways waiting to get into the next class, which was frequently sold out. Eventually, with a full roster of teachers, a morning-to-evening class schedule, and a huge following, she outgrew the small space in the Actors Institute and created the Molly Fox Studio on West 19th Street in New York, a place that quickly became one of the top aerobics studios in the entire city.

We stayed in touch through the years. I became the dean of the personal training program at Equinox Fitness Clubs, and eventually Molly sold her studio and joined Equinox as creative director of group fitness. By now she had a solid national reputation, not only as a businesswoman (she was the IDEA businessperson of the year, a highly competitive award given to outstanding business owners in the fitness industry), but also as a leader and a creative thinker. Plus—people loved her. She seemed to always have this aura around her of lightness and grace. By now she had abandoned aerobics and begun studying yoga seriously. In true Molly form, within a few short years she became one of the best-known yoga teachers in the country. Although I can't prove this, I believe she is more responsible for bringing yoga into the health club arena than anyone else on the planet. She introduced yoga and meditation classes to Equinox, and, eventually, opened her own highly respected studio in Brooklyn where she not only taught, but also created certification training for yoga instructors that continues to this day.

But here's the thing. Molly is really one of those people who truly deserves the much overused term "special." She has a grace. She has a lightness of being. She is the person you turn to when circumstances seem really crummy and the world looks really dark, because she'll always find a way to make it seem less so. Sometimes she does it with humor. Sometimes just her presence will do it. (Sometimes she'll just bring out one of her beloved little dogs, whose cuteness will crack up just about anyone.) She is always what I like to call "a committed listener." And I think one of the reasons she has been so consistently beloved by students and colleagues over the past 25 years is that she is genuinely interested in people. She's kind. And she cares. It's a pretty winning combination.

In many ways our careers have taken parallel paths. I entered the field of personal training 15 years ago with a master's degree in psychology and a deep, abiding interest in the people I was helping to become healthy. It didn't take me too long to discover that helping people transform their bodies took a lot more than just imparting information on exercise and nutrition. Clients seemed to naturally talk to me, and as I began to specialize in weight loss, I realized that weight loss was a much more complicated endeavor than just cutting out food and exercising (as anyone who has tried to lose weight time and time again can attest to). I went back to school to learn nutrition. Eventually I stopped personal training, and worked exclusively in counseling people on nutrition and health issues. In time, by using my natural inclinations and determining what was needed to produce results, I began to focus on the whole person before me, not just the number of calories consumed.

Molly has always been interested in the whole person. And yoga, for her, has always been about accessing a person's deeper spirit and connectedness to the universe. So when she decided to write a book about using yoga for weight loss and asked me to join the party, I couldn't have been happier. I didn't know much about yoga—except for what I've learned from Molly—but I do know a lot about human behavior, personal transformation, commitment, and motivation. And Molly and I share the same vision of how transforming your body—and your health—can transform your life.

I hope that by the time you finish this book, you will come to share our vision.

Introducing Jonny Bowden (by Molly Fox)

I don't know any nutritionist in America who is better at what he does than Jonny Bowden. I'm not saying there aren't any—just that I've never met them!

In the last couple of decades, while I was graduating from aerobics to yoga and working on my own personal journey, Jonny was graduating from the gym world of personal training and moving into the much bigger arena of counseling people on their nutrition, their health, and in some ways—though he would never say this—on their lives. We always stayed in touch, and though we didn't talk that frequently, when we did we would have long discussions not only about exercise and nutrition, but also about the universe, the human spirit, and our own personal transformations and journeys (and, of course, our animals!).

In the 1990s, Jonny was hired by i-Village.com (probably the most famous and successful destination site on the Internet catering to women) to write the Weight Loss Coach column. He fairly quickly gained a national profile both for his amazingly compassionate and humanitarian advice to women regarding weight and body image and for his enormous breadth of knowledge in nutrition and health. (He also gained some notoriety for taking on whole segments of the medical profession and for skewering conservative forces like the American Dietetic Association for what he felt were outdated and irrelevant views on human nutrition, health, and weight—but that's another story!) His Shape-Up program on i-Village was a combination of nutrition, exercise, and self-discovery, and was one of the first I had ever seen that actually took into account the whole person in its approach to weight loss. The program became a book (Jonny Bowden's *Shape Up! The Eight Week Program to Transform Your Body, Your Health and Your Life,* Perseus, 2001) whose motto could very well have been "Come for the weight loss—but stay for the transformation." It's my motto as well.

Jonny went on to have a terrific radio show, and I became his very first guest. We talked about the difference between "getting fit" when you were 20 and getting fit when you were 40 or over. Different priorities, different needs, different lifestyles, and most important, different people—older and wiser and complete with yearnings that went way beyond looking good in the latest midriff-baring T-shirt.

Our conversation leads us to this book. The pages that follow not only address the immediate issue of weight loss and exercise, but also the concerns we see among our client population—people who want to feel better about themselves, their bodies, their relationships, their connectedness to their communities and their world, and ultimately their spirit.

For the sake of consistency in the book, the "voice" you will hear will be mine, except when noted. The meditation, mindful eating, and food journaling exercises were created by both of us and came out of the personal growth work we have done with clients in areas that we believed most influenced their relationships to food and to their bodies.

We hope you enjoy the journey. Come for the weight loss—but stay for the transformation!

Preface
Molly's Story

I started dancing when I was six.

I loved the music and the sweeping strokes the human body can make as it expresses itself. That was my initiation into dance. It began with the pure delight of movement. I was dancing for the pure joy of it.

In the beginning of the fitness movement I started teaching at the Jane Fonda Workout in San Francisco. It was wild. It was the beginning of an era. You could feel the excitement and the energy everywhere. The nascent fitness industry was being born. It was the dawn of a new day. We used to do 12 minutes of aerobics barefoot (this was before the days when Reebok was a household brand name). We played our 12-inch records (remember those?) and were intoxicated by the fact that we could actually do this wild, exciting, and energizing movement in public. Bless you, Jane Fonda.

I was in love with this idea of movement to music. I moved to New York City and fulfilled a dream that had begun when I first started teaching: I opened my own aerobic studio (the Molly Fox Studios). It was a huge success. I won awards, I published books, I made videos. The whole West Coast aerobics thing was really catching on. "No pain, no gain" was the catchphrase of the moment, spandex the outfit du jour. Dance aerobics morphed into step; step evolved into bodyshaping; bodyshaping into weights; then machines; and on and on. There was high-impact and low-impact and later, spinning and cardio-kickboxing. There were classes for every taste and style.

But somewhere in all of this, at least for me, the joy of movement was forgotten. I became lost in the numbers: How many calories was I burning? Where was my heart rate? Was I in my "fat-burning" zone?

Sound familiar?

Then I burned out. It didn't happen all at once, but gradually, over time, I lost my enthusiasm, passion, and love. My body was broken but, more important, so was my spirit. My body no longer seemed to be my friend, an ally in this joyous activity I had once loved. I always hurt—my hips and back were in chronic pain. I began to resent what I did for a living.

I wondered if any of my students were feeling the same way about their exercise programs.

One day I wandered into the Jivamukti Yoga Center in New York City and took my very first yoga class. I'm not sure what propelled me into that place; maybe it was fate, or the universe sending me a message, but I'll never forget the feeling I had: It was as if I had come home. I stayed and became a regular. Not only did my body start to heal, but so did my soul. I felt like I had walked into a whole new world where I could befriend my body again. There was a freedom and a depth of awareness in yoga that would hold and inspire me for years to come. It still does. I had found a place where not only I could transform my body, but where my spirit would sing.

And so began my lifelong love affair with yoga.

Ever since I can remember I was in the 90th percentile of maximum height and weight. That stuck with me and had a strong influence over my body image. I struggled with eating disorders, overexercising, and self-inflicted pain brought on by not accepting what God had given me: a perfectly amazing body capable of so much. The practice of yoga has helped me move for the love of moving again, and to celebrate my unique and special human animal body. My weight may go up and down, but my acceptance of my body's amazing potential and my own humanness—being perfectly imperfect—gives me the freedom to love my body unconditionally.

Over the years, I have lost weight slowly and effortlessly. The acceptance of my body that I experienced through my practice of yoga gave me the inspiration to begin to really see my body as a temple, and to treat it accordingly. We often hear from clients who are distressed because they have "lost their motivation." But I have found that "motivation" isn't necessarily something you "get" or "lose." Rather, it develops, and for me it developed out of the very experiences that I got in my yoga practice. The sense of deep admiration for my human physical potential engendered in me the motivation I had often looked for "outside" of myself—motivation to stay on track with my diet and food choices, to continue practicing, to continue choosing joy, life, and health. When that happens, I have discovered, weight loss is much more effortless.

I came to understand that I was more than just a machine that consumed and burned calories. I realized that I am a spirit body in a human form. I came to believe that love, compassion, and forgiveness were essential ingredients to a healthy, well-balanced life. I learned to forgive myself for the past—including all the times I had overeaten, overexercised, starved myself, or otherwise mistreated the body I had now come to love. Although I am far from perfect and consider myself—and my body—a work in progress, I have come to be in touch with the infinite spirit inside me that reminds me daily that I am not just my body. My breath and my spirit are connected to the Universal.

Our bodies, minds, and spirits are made up of the stuff of God. In that knowledge, I reside.

—Molly Fox

Introduction
Can I Lose Weight Practicing Yoga?

If your mind is empty, it is already ready for anything; it is open to everything. In the beginner's mind there are many possibilities; in the expert's mind there are few.

—Shunryu Suzuki, *Zen Mind, Beginner's Mind*

Can I really lose weight practicing yoga?

This was the question on Ann's mind when she approached Molly at the local coffee emporium one day. Ann had put on weight during two pregnancies, and had never been able to take it off. Her busy work schedule and relationship with her husband left her little time for herself. With two small children in the house she found herself less careful about what she ate, and slowly but surely her weight had ballooned until she no longer felt good about herself. Her stress levels were high and she felt that her health was suffering. "Is it possible," she asked Molly, "that yoga could help me lose weight?"

And the answer, ladies and gentlemen, is . . .

Yes.

Yoga has a well-deserved reputation for gentleness, but many people don't realize how powerfully it can transform the body. Even more important, yoga can change how you practice your daily activities. Did you know that you can practice yoga while on the treadmill? You can!

Below are just a few of the things yoga can do for you:

▥ Tone your muscles.
▥ Increase your stamina.
▥ Give you more focus.

⫶ Reduce your stress.
⫶ Increase your flexibility.
⫶ Change the way your body looks.
⫶ Change the way you look at your body.

Truth be told: Yoga can change your life.

And while dozens of exercise fads will come and go—both of us have seen more than our share during our combined years in the fitness and health business—yoga has been around for more than 2,000 years. It's a system that never gets old or stale and one that you'll never outgrow. In fact, some of yoga's most amazing practitioners are in their eighties. And instead of taking away the pleasure of eating, this weight loss program adds some additional rewards to your life: it relaxes and energizes you while also helping you become thinner and feel better about yourself. The yoga plan presented here can serve as the basis of a practice you can continue for the rest of your life.

A Success Story: The Case of Joan

Joan, a manufacturer's rep in New York City, changed her body and her life when she took up yoga a couple of years ago.

Joan, who stands five-foot-three, wore a dress size of two to four before she was married. During the 12 years of her unhappy marriage, her weight ballooned. Then, after she left her husband, she fell into a deep depression and continued to overeat. "I was divorced, depressed, and a size 16. I hated taking antidepressants, and my therapist wasn't helping me feel better," recalls Joan, who is now in her early forties.

A friend suggested that she take yoga classes twice a week. "I couldn't do anything in the beginning. Every pose was strange to me," Joan recalls. But within four months, the classes had become such a habit that she felt off-kilter when she had to miss one. "When I walked into a class, I felt like I was doing homework, but by the end I always felt relaxed and peaceful," Joan says. The effects of the yoga began carrying over into the rest of her life. When she caught herself worrying—her major leisure-time activity—she would breathe deeply and release the tension. Her days became much less stressful. Joan's depression gradually lifted, and she was filled with newfound energy.

At around the six-month mark, Joan realized that, without taking up any other kind of exercise or consciously changing her eating habits, she was growing thinner. By the end of her first year, she'd gone down to a size six and lost 24 pounds, a weight and size at which she has since remained. These days, she has a new boyfriend and leads a much happier life. Concludes Joan: "Yoga helped me reach the peaceful center in life that made me strong."

Yoga can do the same thing for you. However, you will have an added advantage that Joan did not have: the Yoga Weight Loss Eating Plan, which we will discuss at length in Part 3. Although there are some lucky individuals who can lose weight simply by adding exercise into their daily routines, most long-term research indicates that exercise alone, without a change in diet, is not effective for a large number of people. Combining exercise—such as the routines you will learn in this book—with the sensible changes in your diet that you will also learn here, however, is a winning formula for weight loss. And the sense of centering and expanded awareness of both your body and your spirit that comes with practicing yoga vastly increases the odds that you will not only be successful in losing the weight you want to lose, but in keeping it off as well.

What Does the Research Say?

According to *Time* magazine (April, 2001), 15 million Americans do some kind of yoga in their fitness regimen, and three-quarters of all U.S. health clubs offer classes in yoga. It's the exercise of choice for a huge number of high-profile superstars, none of whom are exactly out of shape: Madonna, Sting, Julia Louis-Dreyfus, Jane Fonda, Angelina Jolie—who used it to get in top shape for her *Tomb Raider* role—Julia Roberts, Gwyneth Paltrow, David Duchovny, all three Dixie Chicks, sports legend Kareem Abdul-Jabbar, Christie Turlington, Meg Ryan, and dozens and dozens of others. Hollywood bad boy Charlie Sheen used a combination of yoga exercises and diet—a program very similar to ours in philosophy—to shed 30 pounds! Looking around at the evidence before your eyes, it would sure appear that these folks are onto something. But what does the science say?

Well, prior to about 20 years ago, not much. Though yoga has been around for several thousand years, it wasn't studied seriously and scientifically until relatively recently. Now, a search on the Web site of the National Library of Medicine turns up no fewer than 628 articles investigating yoga's effect on everything from stress reduction to pulmonary function to hypertension.

According to Dr. Mehmet Oz, one of the foremost leaders in complementary medicine and a cardiac surgeon at New York Presbyterian Hospital in Manhattan, yoga massages the lymph system, promoting draining of the lymph, a fluid made of cellular garbage and waste materials plus important white blood cells. In fact, *The Fat Flush Fitness Program,* a recent book by fitness guru Joanie Greggains and nutrition expert Ann Louise Gittleman, takes the position that moving the lymph through the body is one of the most effective things you can do for weight loss.

Dr. C. Noel Bairey Merz, the director of the Preventive and Rehabilitative Cardiac Center of the famed Cedars Sinai Medical Center in Los Angeles, says the patients at his center who practice yoga show "tremendous benefits"—not the least of which is increased cardiovascular circulation, essential for effective exercise. And Dr. Robert Rose, executive director at the MacArthur Foundation's initiative on mind, brain, body, and health research, says, "Thousands of research studies have shown that in the practice of yoga a person can learn to control such physiologic parameters as blood pressure, heart rate, respiratory function, metabolic rate, skin resistance, brain waves and body temperature, among other body functions."

But what does this mean for weight loss? Can yoga really help you shed pounds?

There are no direct studies on the effect of yoga on weight loss. But there are many that tell us about yoga's impact on the parameters that are absolutely essential to weight loss. For example, an article in the *Journal of Alternative and Complementary Medicine* (1997) stated that after four short weeks of intensive yoga practice, subjects were able to increase their maximum energy output by 21 percent without a significant change in heart rate, showing that yoga had had a decided effect on their exercise performance. Exercise intensity equals calorie burn, and the subjects in this study were obviously burning far more calories after four weeks of yoga than they were prior to entering the study.

On December 8, 2002, an article in *The Indian Journal of Pharmacology* described how "over the last ten years, a growing number of research studies have shown that the practice of hatha yoga can improve strength and flexibility . . . and may help control such physiological variables as blood pressure, respiration and heart rate, and *metabolic rate to improve overall exercise capacity*" (italics added). As you will learn in the book, the increased muscle mass that comes from strength training always leads to a higher metabolic rate, which translates into more calories—and fat—burned even at rest.

Speaking of metabolism, an article in the *Annals of Nutritional Metabolism* (1992) found that there was an increased calorie-burning effect observed in yoga exercisers that lasted beyond 90 minutes after completion of the exercise, "indicating the role of yoga in energy metabolism." And in an article published in the December 2001 issue of the *Indian Journal of Medical Research,* the authors found that a group practicing hatha yoga exercises performed better than a group performing conventional physical exercise training during the same period.

There's more. Research studies, such as the article in the September/October 2000 issue of *Psychosomatic Medicine,* are finding that there is a connection between stress and weight gain. (More about that connection in Chapter 2.)

And highly respected researchers like Dr. Robert Sapolsky have made careers out of studying the connection between stress and a long list of diseases and conditions. We are now finding out through some groundbreaking research that stress—and the hormones produced in response to it—actually contributes in a significant way to weight gain. Yoga reduces stress, which means that the practice of yoga may therefore have a profound effect on the very hormones that send signals to your body to store fat—particularly around the middle.

So does our Yoga Weight Loss Program help you burn fat? Absolutely! It increases aerobic capacity, strength, and exercise performance, improves metabolism and fat-burning ability, helps lymph drainage, and reduces the levels of stress hormones, making it the perfect way to begin a journey that will not only produce the body you've been longing for, but also give you the tools you need to create a life you love. What more could you possibly ask for than that?

How to Use This Book

Molly Fox's Yoga Weight Loss Program presents a three-part plan. The first part is the introduction to yoga, the second part consists of the exercises, and the third part is the eating plan.

Chapter 1 gives you an overview of what yoga is (and what it is not). We'll tell you a little of its history, including how it came to be popular in America, and why it is different from every other kind of exercise. You will learn about how it can affect body consciousness and weight, and how it can create what we call "present moments" that will help you get more fully in touch with who you really are.

Chapter 2 is about balance. You will learn the five main imbalances leading to weight gain, and how to correct them. In addition, you will learn about the role of stress and stress hormones in weight gain and how your yoga weight loss practice can have a profound impact on the situation.

Chapter 3 is about actually creating a yoga weight loss practice and fitting it into your own life. You will learn how to get clear about your goals and why that is so important to the success of this program. You'll learn how to make an effective plan, walk what we call "the Middle Path," and become more mindful and conscious in the process. In addition, there will be some practical suggestions for deciding when, where, and how you will practice, as well as a discussion of the accessories (such as mats, blocks, and straps) that might make your practice more enjoyable. Finally, you will be asked to begin a journal in which you answer some critical questions about your weight, your body, and your life.

Chapters 4, 5, and 6 are the actual asana routines, the exercises (or poses) that you will be doing in your yoga weight loss program. Chapter 4 focuses on a practice for increased energy, stamina, and vitality, Chapter 5 on strength and muscle building, Chapter 6 on a practice for calm and relaxation. All of these routines are given in both 40-minute and 20-minute versions.

You'll learn about a performance concept we call the "EDGE" and how to work at or near it for maximum results. You'll learn how to release tensions, and how to create joy in your movements and poses.

Chapter 8 explains breathing and meditation practices. There is more discussion of the role of stress in weight gain and why the kind of practice you'll learn in this chapter is so critical to both your mental health and your weight loss efforts.

Chapter 9 is a sample two-week practice put together using the 40- and 20-minute versions of the asana routines you learned in chapters 4, 5, and 6. It can serve as a model for the creation of a practice of your own design.

Chapter 10 begins the Yoga Weight Loss Eating Plan. We will introduce you to the philosophy behind the eating program as well as its goals, and why those goals will help you lose weight and keep it off. You'll learn to identify foods high in sugar (which are a primary culprit in creating fat in your body), and the "rules" of putting together good, healthful weight-loss meals.

In Chapter 11 you will get a two-week menu that you can follow exactly as written, although we encourage you to use it as a guide and to feel free to improvise as you become more familiar with this new way of thinking about food and health. This chapter comes with quick recipes for each dish in the two-week sample menu.

Chapter 12 discusses food journaling, one of the most effective techniques for losing weight and keeping it off. This chapter also includes mindful eating exercises designed both to help you get in touch with behavioral patterns that may be hindering your efforts to lose weight and help you create new ones that support your goals.

In Chapter 13 you will learn our three steps toward fat-melting success and how to use them for maximum benefit, particularly in conjunction with the food journal you will have begun in the previous chapter. You will also learn about basics like calories, carbohydrates, fat, and protein and how they affect your weight loss program.

In Chapter 14 you will learn about using self-hypnosis for weight loss, and you will also discover how to make your very own personal self-hypnosis tape and how to use it in your practice. And in Chapter 15 we share with you one of the best "diet secrets" we've ever found—a technique that's sure to accelerate your progress and keep you at your goal when you get there.

As you can see, the Yoga Weight Loss Program progresses in a certain order. For best results you should follow that order by first developing a yoga practice until it feels like a good fit, and only then trying to consciously change the way you eat. A consistent, comfortable practice of poses (asanas) will develop your sense of focus and discipline and will aid immeasurably in teaching you to eat mindfully. Similarly, the focus and discipline gained while you're working on your diet will help you enormously when you tackle changing your life.

You might take up yoga because you want to lose weight, but the hope is that, through this program, you will achieve a healthy, well-balanced life along the way.

Part One
Getting Started

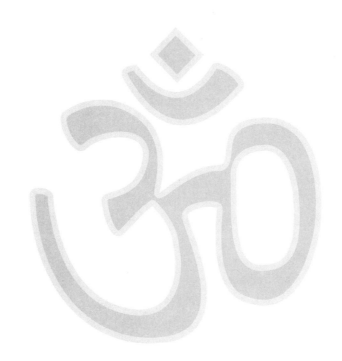

The journey of a
thousand miles begins
with a single step.

—Lao Tzu (father of Taoism)

Chapter One
What Is Yoga?

Our religion keeps reminding
us that we aren't just will and
thoughts. We're also sand and
wind and thunder and rain and
the seasons. All those things.
You learn to respect everything
because you are everything.
If you respect yourself, you
respect all things.

—William Least Heat-Moon,
Native American and author

Yoga. Ask 50 people on the street what it is and you'll probably get
50 different answers. Some will be only dimly aware of yoga as something relating to the weird practices of esoteric holy men dressed in
white robes and headgear. Others may think of it as some kind of
exercise program that stars like Madonna and Sting swear by. Even
those who have actually been exposed to yoga classes may be confused—and no wonder. There are now so many types of yoga out
there that it's hard to tell the players without a scorecard! And that's
not even counting the dozens of crossbreeds like boga (boxing and
yoga), hip-hop yoga, Yoganetics, disco yoga, spin yoga, and yogilates
(a combination of Pilates and yoga)!

Almost unknown in this country until it was first introduced in
1893 at the World Parliament of Religions at the World's Columbian
Exposition in Chicago (the World's Fair), yoga is now one of the
fastest growing popular forms of exercise in America. There is a form
of yoga practice available for virtually every purpose: yoga that is

very physically challenging (Ashtanga, "power yoga" and the like); yoga that focuses on detoxification and general exercise (Bikram); yoga that focuses on precision and alignment (Iyengar); and yoga for meditation or breathing practices. What we will be doing together is a physical practice based on hatha yoga, which will focus on:

- Losing weight
- Burning calories
- Reducing stress
- Creating energy
- Building strength and endurance

But we will also be doing quite a lot more.

You will find yourself creating the ability, both through the yoga poses and the eating program, to have what I call "present moments"—a way of being in the moment that celebrates and honors who you are. And all the while you will be having fun, loving yourself, and learning to appreciate your body's innate abilities.

And guess what? You'll lose weight at the same time! If that sounds like a plan to you, let's get started, define some terms, and get just a touch of historical perspective.

So What Is This Thing Called Yoga, Anyway?

Yoga may be relatively new to the United States, but it is hardly a fad. The practice began two millennia ago in India as a path to self-development and self-realization. Yoga is a unique, ancient system of physical, mental, and spiritual development. Actually, the word *yoga* is the Sanskrit word for union. In its largest context it refers to the union of the individual soul with the collective soul—another way of saying Universal consciousness or God. The original purpose of practicing yoga was to clear away flawed thinking and perception and gain access to a larger, more universal consciousness, bigger than any one person's ego. In fact, the goal of many yoga practitioners was to lose their attachment to ego, which they considered to be the "small self," and find instead an alignment with the "greater self," the self that feels at one with all of humankind. We sometimes get a glimpse of that consciousness when we stare at the ocean, or experience a really peaceful, beautiful moonlit night. It's a sense of wonder at being part of something greater than ourselves, of being connected to something more important than our sometimes petty, everyday concerns. Many people, when they experience this vastness, are moved or overwhelmed by its beauty.

The branch of yoga that most Westerners are familiar with from television and the media is known as hatha yoga. *Ha* means sun and *tha* means moon, so hatha literally means sun/moon, the union of opposites. Another translation is "powerful yoga." Hatha yoga is only one limb of the eight-limbed path of yoga, and one way to enlightenment. It is also the physical aspect of yoga and the path that will help you to lose weight, change your body, and ultimately love your life.

In hatha yoga, physical poses (known as asanas) are used to bring about a sense of harmony or union between the physical individual self and the universe, and to prepare one for meditation. These poses are often based on animal movements and/or parts of nature (for example, see "Downward Facing Dog" in Chapter 4) and they call your entire body into play.

With smooth, gentle movements that are easy on the joints, the actions in yoga stretch muscles while also strengthening them. Newly de-tensed muscles make you feel relaxed and improve your internal energy flow. Newly strengthened muscles boost your metabolic rate, making you more efficient at burning fat. The exercise itself uses up calories. And you become more adept at coping with stress, making it far less likely that you'll turn to food for comfort.

Yoga really made a dent in the popular consciousness when the Beatles first embraced the Indian guru Maharishi Mahesh Yogi, and followed him to Rishikesh, India, in 1968. Maharishi Yogi became "guru to the stars" through his association with the Beatles, and thousands of people in the United States learned his popular technique, Transcendental Meditation. This fascination with all things Indian was a dominant theme in what was then known as the "counterculture," '60s radicals and hippies who embraced lifestyles outside the mainstream and were often in the forefront of cultural trends. But yoga's popularity waned in the early 1980s, coinciding with the surge of interest in much more aggressive forms of exercise such as high-impact aerobics, Jazzercise, and the Jane Fonda Workout.

But in the 1990s yoga reached a whole new audience, this time among a far more mainstream population. Most of these people had grown up thinking of yoga as simply some strange esoteric Indian

The actions in yoga stretch muscles while also strengthening them.

religious practice in which its practitioners, some Indian yogis, could attain enormous physical and mental control. For example, in the 1970s, a certain Swami Rama from the Himalayan mountains stunned the academic community by controlling bodily functions formerly believed to be involuntary. Among other feats, he raised his heart rate from 70 to 300 beats a minute on demand, and caused the temperature of one of his hands to become 10 degrees lower than the other.

These superhuman practices—including lying down on a bed of nails or changing one's blood pressure or heart rate—came out of the Indian culture, where they served very specific spiritual purposes that are beyond the scope of this book.

Most modern-day practitioners, especially in America, have far different goals in mind when taking up yoga. Today the 20 million Americans who practice yoga—more than triple the six million figure of 1994—are looking for peace of mind, better health, stronger muscles, and a better-looking body. The ancient practice has been especially embraced by baby boomers who have grown tired of the "no pain, no gain" philosophy of the '80s and the demands that traditional exercises, like running, place on their knees and other joints. What began as a new trend became a soulful life-shift.

This book offers you both a yoga workout practice that will reshape your body and help you lose weight and an eating plan that will support you in maintaining that new weight for the rest of your life. What makes it different from other exercise plans that promise similar results is that yoga practice does more—it addresses not only the needs of your body, but those of your mind and soul as well. We have taken a very powerful ancient practice and adapted it to your needs today.

Do it mindfully and consciously and you will not only change your body, you will change your entire life.

Being Present in the Moment

The next time you're in the gym, take a look at the exercisers around you: people running on treadmills, riding stationary bikes, or huffing and puffing on the stair climbers. How many have headphones on? How many are staring ahead at the bank of television monitors that line the cardio area in most trendy health clubs? Probably the majority. And there's a simple reason for all of this: They're trying to distract themselves from the effort they're expending and the boredom they're experiencing.

The group fitness classes don't fare much better. The high-pitched, chipmunk-sounding tapes speeded up to jolt everyone's heart rate and the forced whoop-de-wooing of the participants create a frantic, possessed environment that has very little to do with fun, ease, or pleasure. Aerobic and step class mavens preach "the harder the better." As the group bounces and shoots out buckets of sweat, their attention turns outward—almost exclusively on the mirror.

Contrast that to any yoga class, anywhere.

The difference is immediately apparent. Yoga requires attention, mindfulness, and focus. Yoga requires that you be present in the moment.

With yoga, as you move into or hold the various postures, you understand completely what muscular sensation feels like. You are acutely aware of where your various muscles and limbs are and what they're doing at any given moment. Even when you are staying relatively still, you are making subtle adjustments, extending some muscles farther away from your center and bringing others closer to you, all the while breathing deeply and rhythmically. By focusing on your muscles and your breath, you keep your attention fixed on what you're doing at all times. Your mind doesn't get cluttered by thoughts of what is past or future. At any given time as you practice yoga, you are profoundly aware of what it feels like to be you, creating an ability to live in the moment that carries over into your daily life.

While doing yoga, many people go into what's been called a "flow" state, which athletes often refer to by the more flashy phrase "the zone." Flow is exactly what it sounds like—a state in which you are not watching and evaluating yourself, but just being.

Mihaly Csikszentmihalyi, who first popularized the flow concept, defines it as complete absorption in an activity whose challenges mesh perfectly with your abilities. If you've ever played a tennis or golf game when you seemed to hit every shot perfectly without having to stop and "think" about your every move, you know what flow feels like. You're in the midst of a flow experience when you are totally absorbed by what you are doing. You can get the feeling of flow from telling jokes at a party, writing a letter where the words just tumble out onto the page, or even playing a card game with a bunch of friends. The experience is always pleasurable—perhaps even mystical—and could very well be the highlight of your day.

Research on exercisers by exercise scientist Susan A. Jackson and Csikszentmihalyi, published in a book called *Flow in Sports* (Human Kinetics), indicates that the flow state most often occurs when the effort presents a moderate challenge. If what you're doing is too easy—think walking on a treadmill—you get bored and tune out. If it's too difficult, you get anxious. That tennis match against a much-better opponent, a step routine that can't be mastered, a run that's too long—they all create distress. Such uneasiness interferes with an exerciser's ability to attain flow by breaking his or her concentration. But when the challenge suits your abilities, you have a good chance of experiencing flow.

Yoga poses can be modified for people of all levels, so it is easy to find the appropriate degree of challenge for slipping into this state of intense concentration. Many people who consistently do yoga find that they experience flow more and more often throughout the day—one reason yoga has a reputation for giving people "bliss."

Movement, Body Consciousness, and Weight Loss

So the take-home point is this: Yoga is about much more than just the body; it is about beauty (inner and outer) and spirit and soul. The first step in weight loss is acceptance of what is. This doesn't mean you have to "settle" for the way things are now, just that you have to accept where you are first, in order to create space to move on and create something new.

The first step in my own weight loss was to give thanks for the fact that I had a beautiful and capable body, even if it didn't look exactly as I would have liked it to look. Accomplishing this can be hard sometimes, especially when you have spent years feeling shame or embarrassment about being "overweight." But to move on, you must take that first step of acceptance. You have to accept that you are whole and complete right now, exactly the way things are. Stand up and say "I rock!" Bring the largeness of who you really are in spirit to your practice, "lighten up," and get ready to enjoy the process. Join me in one of the best ways in the world to lose weight and learn to love yourself at the same time!

Look, I have always been interested in what I call the "consciousness" of movement. Even back in the heyday of the fitness movement

When everyone was running around frantically doing aerobic and high-impact step classes, even with all the great disco music whirling around throngs of people and thongs of spandex, I was always looking for the integrity of the exercise. This doesn't mean that I wasn't having fun. It's just that I was looking for something that connected my joy in moving my body to the joy in my soul. For me they were not separate things.

When I found yoga, I felt like I had come home. I had always loved moving my body, from the time I was a child. Now I had found a way to not only make that movement feel good, but to be meaningful as well.

Many people speak about the spiritual connection they feel when they practice yoga. For me that spirituality comes from the moment-to-moment conscious connection I have with my body when I practice. I love the way my body feels when it stretches, when it shakes, and sometimes even when it feels the sensation of work or physical challenge. I even love the burn!

But I also love the peace afterwards. I love the gentleness and stillness I feel after I have worked hard. I love the sense of accomplishment and progress and change. I celebrate my body and invite you to do the same, with every pose you take on.

The spirit of the original yoga was to unite your day-to-day personality with the deepest part of you that never changes: your wholeness and essential goodness. You see, whether you have 10 pounds to lose—or more than 100—your essential, inner goodness is never changing and is always there if only you can connect with it. You don't have to lose weight to tap into that, and, in fact, it is my experience that if you begin tapping into it right away, you will lose weight faster and with less effort and struggle than you ever thought possible. Even if you are already at a weight that you are happy with and just want to use the program to get in shape, your inner goodness is something solid that you can learn to connect with. It is always present. Unite with it. It is the stuff of contentment and peace.

Love yourself, live your life fully and graciously, move and breathe consciously, and watch the pounds melt away!

When I found yoga, I felt like I had come home.

Chapter Two
Finding Your Balance

I never thought of achievement. I just did what came along for me to do—the thing that gave me the most pleasure.

—Eleanor Roosevelt

Yoga improves balance, both in the physical sense of the word and in the metaphorical sense. Anyone who has ever seen a skilled practitioner hold any of the advanced poses can instantly see the superb amount of control and balance required to master the positions. The yoga asanas build the muscle strength, flexibility, alignment, and body awareness that make it possible for you to, say, bend over while standing on only one leg for several seconds. Because the poses typically use all of the muscles in the body, yoga also builds balanced strength, so that the muscles that must work in tandem (think of the hamstrings in the back of the legs and the quadriceps in the front) maintain the optional ratios of power.

But yoga also develops an inner sense of balance and calm as well. Yoga is traditionally believed to balance out the flow of energy (prana) that flows through the body in seven energy centers, releasing blockages so that you feel revitalized and alive—even "blissful." Probably most important of all for our purposes is the fact that people who study yoga for a significant length of time develop a much more balanced view of their bodies. When you feel your body become open, strong, and stable, when you realize that it's able to perform in ways you didn't dream possible, when you personally experience the meshing of body and spirit that is almost always a part of yoga practice, you appreciate how great your body really is. Whether you're a size 2 or 22, yoga helps you see that your body is really there for you. As one formerly obese man told *Yoga Journal,* "The diet industry has set up millions of Americans to fail. Fortunately you can never fail in yoga, which emphasizes accepting the body as it is."

Balance and Food

When you are unhappy with your weight, you develop a somewhat unbalanced attitude toward food. Food becomes the enemy—cravings become a foreign "thing" that takes over your life, and obsessiveness about food becomes the order of the day. You may forget that food is in fact the stuff of life—and that it can be fun. Far from being an opponent in your life to be "mastered," it is really your ally; it is the fuel that keeps you moving, thinking, talking, and functioning throughout the day. You may forget how much pleasure there can be in eating. Who wants to think of life without a perfectly delicious piece of dark chocolate every now and again? Who wants to go through life on one nonstop, deprivation-based diet after another?

Your eating habits become problematic when your desire for food is out of balance with what your body truly needs to function optimally. Burn up more calories than you consume and you lose weight. Take in more calories than you burn up and—you know all too well what the consequences are. You can see the results every day on your butt, thighs, and waistline.

This equation of calories in and calories out is made a bit more complicated by the fact that not everyone uses calories at the same rate. Some people process calories very efficiently; think about your friend who seems to be able to eat anything she wants without gaining a pound. Most of us are not so lucky. People who have what is called "slow" metabolisms tend to burn up calories sluggishly and economically; there is often a lot left over to turn to fat. These slower metabolisms were once very adaptive for the human animal. In times of famine, the ability to store fat easily kept our ancestors alive through the frequently harsh times when food was scarce.

The problem is, we've got Fred Flintstone genes in a George Jetson world. Our ability to hold on to calories and store fat easily is no longer an asset in a world of food courts, convenience stores, and super-sizing. A "slow" metabolism that may have once saved us from starvation by making it easy to store fat now hastens our chances of dying from one of the many conditions, such as heart disease and diabetes, that are linked to obesity.

The key to losing weight is manipulating three variables—calories in, calories out, and your metabolic rate. If you want to slim down you need to eat less, burn more calories, and/or push your metabolic rate to a higher level. But here's where it gets tricky. Eat too little and your metabolic rate will slow down. Your body thinks it's starving, so it turns down your internal thermostat, learning to survive on less food. The result? You stop losing weight even though you're eating practically nothing. And when you go back to normal eating, your body holds on to all those calories for dear life, thinking it needs to store them for the next emergency. This is the well-known rebound or yo-yo effect seen in those who live from diet to diet.

So once again we see that the answer lies in balance. To achieve the results you want to achieve, you need to rectify various imbalances in your life—for example, finding the balance between eating too much (fat storage) and eating too little (fat conservation!). You need to do this without starving yourself and without exercising at a maniacal intensity. Here's how our program helps solve the most common imbalances.

Imbalance Number #1: Your Metabolism Has Slowed Down

Your parents probably got heavier as they entered their senior years, and your grandparents probably did, too. Before rampant obesity became a public health concern in the United States, and before the era when baby boomers with their fitness consciousness reached middle age and decided that they didn't have to get fat, most Americans accepted what they thought was a basic fact of life: They'd get fatter as they got older. Their metabolic rate would "slow down."

We now know that "fact" is far from inevitable.

Most people, as they age, become less active. When you stop using muscles, those muscles begin to atrophy. Since muscle is the place where most of your calories are burned, the loss of muscle inevitably leads to the loss of calorie-burning ability. By not exercising your muscles, you slowly lose the most effective fat-burning "furnaces" in the body. Hence, the well-known phenomenon of a slowed-down metabolism. Muscle doesn't "turn to fat" (they are two separate tissues), but as you lose muscle it becomes very easy to put on fat. And that's exactly what happens when you don't exercise your muscles in a rigorous way. You simply don't have the same fat-burning ability you had when you were younger and had more muscle.

Here's the deal: The bulk of the calories you take in each day are used up in maintaining your organs, such as your brain, kidney, liver and muscles. A woman who is five-foot-four and weighs 132 pounds, for instance, might typically burn about 1,300 calories a day at rest, if she did nothing more than sleep all day. That's what's known as her "resting metabolic rate." Add another 300 or so calories for "walking around" and she's up to 1,600 for the day. But if a high percentage of her 132 pounds is body fat, she may not need 1,600 calories to maintain her weight. Since muscle is the main "consumer" of calories—fat takes almost no calories to maintain—and since she doesn't have much muscle, if she eats the 1,600 or so calories you would predict she needs, she'll actually gain weight because she's taking in more than her body requires.

But here's the good news: Change her body composition so that she's got more muscle, and her caloric needs go up. Her body's ability to burn fat will be restored and she will turn into a lean, calorie-burning machine.

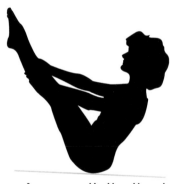

Any activity that increases your muscle mass **also boosts your resting metabolic rate.**

Want more good news? Any activity that increases your muscle mass also boosts your resting metabolic rate, making it easier to achieve your ideal weight. In the July 12, 2001, issue of *USA Today,* Nanci Hellmich reported on a recent study done at the University of Maryland in which participants raised their metabolic rate by about 7 percent after working out with weights. Other studies have shown similar results. Building strong muscles is such an effective way to lose weight that some personal trainers—whose livelihood depends on producing results—tell their clients to forget about emphasizing aerobics and to concentrate instead on strength training. "Strength training is critical for people with a weight-control problem," says Miriam Nelson, director of the Center for Physical Fitness at Tufts

University in Boston. And Wayne Wescott, Ph.D., a highly respected exercise physiologist and coauthor of *Specialized Strength Training* adds, "If you are only doing aerobics, you are missing the boat. You will lose muscle mass and your metabolism will slow down as you age if you don't strength train."

Many yoga poses—especially the standing ones—efficiently strengthen muscles, and in such a gentle way that you won't be sore the next day. The muscle-building routine presented in Chapter 5 emphasizes asanas that tone you up and help boost your metabolic rate. Remember that lean muscle is very much like the engine in a car. Just as a bigger engine burns more gas, bigger muscles burn more calories. The strength routines in the Yoga Weight Loss Program are designed to improve the ratio of your lean muscle to body fat, setting up a more favorable environment for calorie burning, and ultimately revving up your metabolism.

Imbalance #2: You Don't Exercise Enough

Ever visit Europe and wonder why most Europeans don't seem to be as fat as Americans, even though they eat just as many fatty foods? One reason is that they walk everywhere! In a recent study, researchers used pedometers to measure the number of steps taken daily by representative groups in middle America and in France. They found that the French walked almost three times more than the Americans on a daily basis.

Years ago, Americans groomed their lawns with rotary mowers, washed laundry by hand, and actually walked to places like work and church. Believe it or not, at one point we had televisions without remote controls and had to actually get up and walk to the set every time we wanted to change the channel (yup, those calories do count and they do add up). British researchers have estimated that in the nineteenth century, before the explosion of obesity in the Western world, people burned up about 800 more calories a day than they do now.

For many people, a key strategy for losing weight is to burn off extra calories each day by exercising. In fact, research from the National Weight Control Registry looked at the habits of people who have successfully lost weight (defined as a minimum of 30 pounds kept off for at least one year, though the average amount of weight lost was 60 pounds, and it was kept off for five years!). Though the methods that the 3,000 participants originally used to lose weight varied considerably, those who kept it off were found to have several habits in common. Hands down, the most important habit the "weight loss winners" shared was exercise, which helped them burn about 2,700 calories per week.

A recent study in *Medicine and Science in Sports and Exercise* (2001) by Jakicic, Clark, and Associates entitled "Appropriate Intervention Strategies for Weight Loss and Prevention of Weight Regain for Adults" confirmed the importance of regular exercise in maintaining weight loss and preventing the rebound effect. (We have observed this to be true time and time again in our experience with clients.) The other habit of those who lost weight successfully was self-monitoring, often by keeping a food diary. We'll discuss this at length in Chapter 12.

Without a doubt, the form of activity that burns the most calories is aerobic exercise. Aerobic simply means "with oxygen." You are using your aerobic energy system right now, as you're reading this book. You're just not taxing it very strenuously. Those heart-thumping, shin-pounding workouts that were known in the 1980s as "aerobics classes" simply put more demand on your body's ability to deliver oxygen to the lungs and muscles than, for example, walking does, but walking is still very much an "aerobic" exercise, as is the Yoga Weight Loss Program. Activities like aerobics classes and running, however, come with a price tag. The hard impact of the feet on the ground puts continuous strain on the exerciser's joints (particularly the knees and back), and few people over the age of 40 are truly comfortable with high-impact aerobics classes. Also, many people, regardless of age, simply don't enjoy the experience of total exhaustion that can come with hard aerobic activities.

Yoga, like walking, provides a low-impact aerobic routine that is easy to sustain for 45 minutes or more, and burns a substantial amount of calories in the bargain. When you move quickly in a flowing fashion between a series of postures—a technique often known as power yoga—the yoga workout raises your heart rate effectively without making you feel drained and listless. In Chapter 4 you'll find a calorie-burning routine that will increase the number of calories you expend in a day.

We're now finding out through excellent research (notably, Peeke and Chrousos, 1995, "Hypercortisolism and Obesity") that stress can cause weight gain, particularly in the abdominal area. Stress eating actually has a physiological basis. It's not "all in your mind." Here's how it works.

Nature gave us the phenomenal ability to go "on alert" almost instantly when presented with a threat. What happens is that the two small, walnut-shaped glands called the adrenals (which sit on top of your kidneys) send out hormones, such as adrenaline and cortisol, that are released whenever the body senses that action is needed immediately. This system served to protect our Paleolithic ancestors from such dangers as woolly mammoths. The release of these hormones sends sugar into the bloodstream to be transformed into the energy needed to either pick up a club and fight or run up a tree—which is why these are called the "fight or flight" hormones.

You have probably experienced the feeling of a surge of adrenaline if you've ever had to slam on the brakes of your car to avoid an accident, or if you've ever felt unfamiliar footsteps approaching you from behind on a dark street. These hormones are necessary for existence—without them we'd perish. The problem is this: They were meant as a kind of emergency signaling system, which wasn't meant to run all the time. Nature never anticipated lifestyles in which we would be constantly under the gun at work, stuck in traffic, talking on the phone while trying to grab something to eat, dealing with emergencies with the kids, and trying to make a deadline at the office—frequently all in the same day. Our stress hormones are running on overload. The situation is made worse by the two main pillars of stress: dieting and lack of sleep.

What does this all have to do with weight? Well, Peeke and Chrousos showed that elevated levels of the stress hormone cortisol lead to weight gain, particularly around the midsection. They wanted to determine why stress leads to overeating, which then leads to fat being deposited deep inside the abdominal area. So they decided to look at a rare medical condition called Cushing's Syndrome, a disease brought about by prolonged exposure to large amounts of the stress hormone cortisol. The usual cause of this condition is a tiny tumor either in the brain or the adrenal glands (or once in a while in other organs, such as the lungs). This tumor makes the body produce high levels of cortisol which, in turn, makes the patient very sick. People with Cushing's Syndrome have an apple-shaped body because of the large amount of fat accumulated in the belly. Peeke and Chrousos picked Cushing's Syndrome to study because it basically imitates what would happen if we walked around with chronically elevated levels of cortisol for months or years at a time without knowing it.

And here's what happens: The chronically high levels of cortisol stimulate cells to continually store more fat. This in turn leads to a large accumulation of intra-abdominal fat, which Peeke refers to as Toxic Weight., This fat, because of its location in the central abdominal region, is particularly dangerous. Many studies have found that central abdominal fat—more so than fat in any other part of the body—is correlated with a number of serious medical illnesses such as heart disease. Stress can, as Peeke points out, literally change the shape of your body! In other words, stress can make you fat (and fat in the most dangerous places of all!).

The thinking goes like this: When the body is in a state of emergency, it sends a message to the brain to refuel. And the fastest source of energy for refueling is sugar—that's the physiological basis behind those carbohydrate cravings at times of stress. We store that "stress fat" around our midsections because it is more easily mobilized there when it's needed for the next emergency. (Women will often store it in the hips, butt, and thighs before menopause; the logic is that nature knows that women need their "middle" for pregnancy. After menopause, women often store their fat in the same place as men.)

Even women who are not overweight but are vulnerable to the effects of stress and the stress hormone cortisol are likely to have higher levels of abdominal fat, according to recent studies at Yale University. Elissa S. Epel, Ph.D., led an investigation of the connection between stress and fat, published in the September/October 2000 issue of *Psychosomatic Medicine.* She found that "women with greater abdominal fat had far more negative moods and higher levels of life stress. Greater exposure to life stress or psychological vulnerability to stress may explain their enhanced [levels of cortisol]. In turn, their cortisol exposure may have led them to accumulate greater abdominal fat."

Cortisol, like all hormones, also sends a "message" of its own to the body: "Keep the fat for emergency, burn the muscle tissue for fuel." We've already learned that muscle is your most important ally in the fight against fat, so the loss of muscle through the action of cortisol further slows down your metabolism, thereby making it even harder to lose weight. Nutritionist Michael Colgan once called cortisol "the Grinch of bodybuilding" for this very reason—it tears down muscle. And we haven't even mentioned the aging effect of cortisol on other organs in the body, specifically the brain!

The obvious conclusion: Stress is the natural enemy of fat loss. Yet it's a constant fact of modern life. What to do? This weight loss program is the perfect answer to this modern-day imbalance.

When faced with stress, some people reach for a cigarette, some for a drink, some for food, some for all three. The feeling of being under stress is intensely uncomfortable for many people, and our first response is often to evade those edgy sensations through unhealthy habits.

Yoga presents a much more positive approach. It is indisputable that the consistent practice of yoga is highly effective both in lowering our baseline feelings of stress and in helping us cope with specific distressful moments.

How does the Yoga Weight Loss Program reduce stress? Well, it happens in a variety of ways. Because the program demands strong concentration, it gives us a break from anxiety-producing thoughts; sometimes a rest is all we need to get back in gear. At the same time, stretching movements release muscle tension and energy blocks, helping us relax for hours afterwards. Also, the slow, deep breathing used in yoga has long been used to create a sense of calm. A recent study cited in the December 22, 2001, issue of the *British Medical Journal* found out why: This kind of practice brings our breathing in sync with certain rhythmic fluctuations in the way blood flows throughout our bodies. The synchronicity is intensely soothing, like being rocked in a cradle or like lying next to a purring cat. The *Journal* article concluded that the yoga mantras given to the study participants induced "favorable psychological and possibly physiological effects." No wonder, then, that some people leave yoga classes feeling as if they've just gotten up from a deep, refreshing sleep.

For many people, a reduction in stress means they have fewer urges to overeat. California acupressure/yoga expert Michael Reed Gach notes that many people mistake tension in their stomachs for the sensation of hunger, and try to reduce that unpleasant feeling by

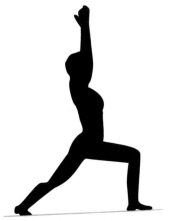

The slow, deep breathing used in yoga has long been used to create a sense of calm.

eating. He believes that postures that put pressure on certain spots in the stomach—an example would be the Boat Hold poses described in Chapter 5—are especially useful for relieving this tension and therefore feelings of hunger. But all yoga postures help reduce stress and thus reduce the urge to overeat. Chapter 6 presents a stress-reducing routine that focuses on relaxation.

Imbalance #4: You Eat Without Realizing It

Earlier, we mentioned two things that predict success in weight loss. One of them is consistent exercise. Can you recall the other one?

Give up? It's a food diary! That's right, keeping a food diary (here-after known as a journal) has proven to be the most consistent predictor of success in the weight loss game. Why? Because lack of awareness is the enemy of weight loss, and a food journal keeps us honest. Most of us eat in a semiconscious state. How often have you found yourself staring at an open refrigerator, just munching on what-ever seemed to beckon? Or wandering at a buffet dinner while engaged in animated conversation, sampling bits and pieces of every-thing on the table? Or reaching for a second and third helping at the dinner table "just because it was there"? We're all guilty of these behaviors, and they contribute mightily to our expanding waistlines.

It's pretty obvious why exercise might make a difference in this scenario, and why consistent exercise might be one of the best pre-dictors of success in keeping weight off. But why the food journal? To illustrate, let's move away a bit from the discussion of food and weight and take a slight digression into the field of money (right up there with weight in its anxiety-causing ability!). The connection will be obvious soon enough.

Years ago, Jonny went to see a well-known financial planner in New York City named Stephen Pollan. Pollan had written a number of interesting and controversial books, including *Die Broke,* and was developing something of a reputation as a "life coach" for his ability—similar to that of the well-known financial commentator Suzie Orman—to tie issues of money management into greater life themes. He (like Orman) had realized early on that the way people manage money often is a window into many more personal issues, conflicts, and life themes, and that managing money effectively is rarely simply a matter of getting better information—there are simply too many emotional issues involved, and you will never get the job done if you ignore them. (Perhaps you're already beginning to see a connection to food and exercise? If not, read on.)

Anyway, Pollan had an interesting approach to creating a budget that involved the following assignment, which he was ruthless in enforcing. He required you to keep a diary of every penny that you spent for two weeks. Not only that, but you had to journal every single ATM withdrawal you made, and where the money from those withdrawals went. Sounds simple, right?

Jonny immediately recognized a parallel to his own work with weight loss clients, and mentioned it to Pollan. He added that his weight loss clients tended to hate doing the food journal, and asked Pollan if he had had the same experience with his financial management clients when it came to doing the money journal. Pollan quickly replied that keeping the money diary—particularly the ATM receipts and accounting—was undoubtedly the most hated and resisted part of his program. People basically went nuts trying to avoid it. Why? Because most people, especially those who are having trouble managing money (or food), live in a state of unconsciousness about it. How many ATM receipts can you account for right now? Do you know where that last $20 (or $100) withdrawal went? Jonny certainly didn't, and according to Pollan, neither did any of his clients. And people resisted keeping track of it because it forced them to be conscious and accountable for spending in a way that they were not accustomed to and wished to avoid.

And so it is with food. Jonny, who has been doing weight management and dietary counseling for years, has found in client after client an almost rigid resistance to the assignment of keeping an accurate, day-by-day, meal-by-meal food journal. The most usual response: "Oh, I can tell you pretty much what I ate yesterday." Or: "I eat the same thing every day." Or: "Let me see—I eat a lot of chicken, broccoli . . . hmmm . . . once in a while some eggs. Don't like sweets much." Basically all of us—whether clients of a weight management specialist or a money management specialist—do not want to shine a 1,000-watt flashlight on our most unconscious and unexamined habits, which are the same ones that got us into the predicament we need help with in the first place! We like our habits, we like being unconscious, and we like not examining our lifestyle choices too closely. We prefer to simply coast through our lives without too much examination, only to find that the very choices that we make every day—and believe it, they are choices, even if we don't think about them carefully—be they about food, exercise, money, or time management, are returning to bite us in the proverbial, ever-expanding butt!

So the food journal is a way of enforcing consciousness in a particular area of our life that is having a profound effect not only on our waistlines but on our health in general. Without knowing where we are starting, it is very difficult to know what changes to make, and virtually impossible to tell if those changes are making any difference. The food journal is actually empowering. It is only by looking at something head on, without fear and trembling, without anxiety and shame, that we can address it the way it needs to be addressed: with mindfulness, care, and determination. The food journal is an important tool to help you craft a new relationship with food. If you follow through, you will lose weight, keep it off, and change the way you feel about your body and your life.

In the end, the food journal, the eating program, and especially the yoga routines you will learn in this book are all about mindfulness.

The longer you practice yoga, the better you become at staying focused on what you're doing. This mindfulness has the effect of making moments seem bigger. Without the noise of your internal monologues and the distractions caused by multitasking, experiences seem more intense and enjoyable.

Mindfulness is an especially important habit to develop if you're concerned about your weight, which is where the use of the food journal can really help. When we don't pay attention to what we're eating, we miss the internal cues that our bodies send out to tell us that we've had enough. We end up consuming a lot of calories without either noticing or enjoying them. And the risk is especially great when you are doing something else, such as watching television or cooking dinner.

At least a dozen studies since 1985 have established a significant correlation between television watching and risk of obesity. Most recently, in the April 9, 2003, edition of the *Journal of the American Medical Association,* Hu, Li, Colditz, Willett, and Manson published an article in which they stated that sedentary behaviors—especially television watching—were significantly associated with risk of obesity and type 2 diabetes.

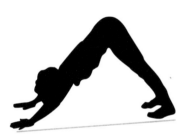

Mindfulness is an especially important habit to develop if you're concerned about your weight.

Many other published papers and studies confirm this belief, including a 1996 article on the link between children and obesity in the *Archives of Pediatrics and Adolescent Medicine* (Gortmaker and colleagues) and a 1991 article on television viewing and obesity in adult females in the *American Journal of Public Health* (Tucker and Bagwell). The evidence is incontrovertible: Watching television is directly correlated with eating more than you should, and it may well be due to the semiconscious state we're in when we stare at the tube and nibble mindlessly. (It may also have to do with the approximately 90,000 commercials for food products that the average consumer is exposed to yearly—but that's another story!)

In Chapter 12, we will show you how to apply the mindfulness developed in your yoga practice to your eating habits through the use of journaling.

Imbalance #5: You Fill Empty Spots in Your Life with Food

Going hand in hand with unconscious eating is the tendency many people have to eat for emotional reasons. In several ways, our bodies serve as metaphors for the state of our lives. Many of us visibly carry around our sense of burden, giving us a stooped, overwhelmed posture. Often you can see it in our choice of language: We "shoulder" responsibilities when we must get something done; and we "dig in our heels" or "stand our ground" when we don't want to budge on something. And when we are "hungry"—for love, acceptance, success, whatever—we open the refrigerator. For many people, an empty life feels like an empty stomach.

Yoga provides a way to fill up that space. In most yoga postures, your muscles move in two directions. Some pull away from your center and others draw back into it. Metaphorically, when you practice yoga, you are learning both to reach out to other people and to draw back into your own strength. This dual action—going outward and going inward—is repeated in the ethical precepts presented in the classic texts by the ancient yoga master Patanjali. These guidelines, such as developing an attitude of gratitude and dealing with people truthfully, form an incredibly useful way to transform your life as you change your waistline. You'll find these guidelines in the Conclusion.

Most of us have many people who depend on us. We have children, spouses, friends, lovers, bosses, family—and on any given day we may feel pulled in many different directions. Those of us who are caretakers by nature often fare badly in these situations because our instinct is to take care of others at the expense of taking care of ourselves. But sometimes even the caretaker needs caretaking. The challenge is to find balance between our responsibilities to others and our responsibility to ourselves.

That's where we might begin. We are responsible for ourselves. Others can love and support us, but ultimately we are responsible for our own happiness, and it is we who will make our lives happy or not, successful or not, and fulfilling or not.

Making yourself the top priority is the key to being whole and also the key to being able to be there fully for others. By taking care of yourself, you are also modeling a way of being that says "I think enough of myself to take care of *me*." Jane was used to spending a couple of hours in the evening overseeing her kids' homework. Deep inside, she felt that if she didn't exercise careful supervision over this task it would never get done and the kids would end up playing video games all night, or talking on the phone or on the Internet. So she took on their homework as her personal burden. When Jane wanted to begin a yoga practice she immediately came up against the issue of time: Where would she get it? The evening seemed the most obvious choice, but then what would her kids do? Would they get their homework done? Would they think she was abandoning them? Would the universe see her as a bad, selfish, uncaring mother?

Jane decided to try a compromise. She would spend half an hour setting her kids up with their homework. She would make it very clear that she was not to be disturbed during the next 40 to 60 minutes while she did her yoga practice. She would then spend the last half hour of the evening with her kids as they wrapped up the homework session. She worked out the bumps, and it turned her conflict into a growth experience for everyone involved. Jane got to take care of herself, do her yoga practice, and see that her kids could be responsible at the same time. The result? A win-win for everyone.

When you do decide to take time for yourself, you will sometimes run into a bit of resistance from families or friends. These well-meaning people have learned to relate to you in a very specific way, possibly in a very specific role. This is a problem many overweight people run into when they ultimately lose weight. Their role in the circle of friends or coworkers as the "fat, jolly girlfriend" or in the family as the "earth mother" is changing, and it often causes subconscious distress for many of the people around them. These folks subtly encourage them to revert back to being the familiar figure they are used to dealing with.

Don't worry. Your family and friends will adjust. Tell them that you love them but in order to give to them fully and completely, you have to become as big and as fully realized a human being as you can be. You love them, but you love yourself too. And right now you are doing what is necessary for your health. That means doing your yoga practice, eating the foods that support your new lifestyle and, ultimately, surrounding yourself with people who truly support you.

Finding a balance between your natural instinct to care for others and your nascent, developing ability to take care of yourself is critical to successfully negotiating your path to a new you. You deserve to have the body you love and feel great and happy at the same time. Every time you take a positive step toward being healthy and happy, it's like depositing money in the bank of life.

Become wealthy with success!

Balancing Yoga with Other Exercise

We're often asked about combining yoga with other kinds of exercise. Many people, for example, come to yoga after being exposed to it in their health club or gym, where classes are often sandwiched in between spinning, bodyshaping, or cardio-kickboxing! They ask us if it is productive to continue with their favorite exercise class while adding yoga to the menu. Others have a long history of training with weights and have gotten good results with this method of exercise. Many of our clients jogged several times a week, or power walked or rode their bikes. Still others, especially in recent years, were devotees of Pilates. And, of course, many people come to yoga as their primary (or only) form of exercise, to get in shape, lose weight, reduce stress, and connect with their spirituality.

So the question becomes: Can I combine yoga with other physical activities? Should I combine yoga with other physical activities for maximum results?

Well the easy answer is this: The more movement, the better. In fact, your yoga practice will only make your other activities more pleasurable, efficient, and effective. Weight training helps to preserve or build muscle, which, as we've pointed out, is your best ally in the journey to lose pounds and inches, because muscle is where your calories are burned. So weight training can be an excellent adjunct to your yoga practice. And cardiovascular activities like jogging, walking, swimming, bike riding, stair climbing, or hiking—aerobic exercise—is great for the heart, the lungs, and the circulatory system, and also releases those feel-good chemicals in the brain, the endorphins.

You can feel confident doing any type of cardiovascular activity on the same day as you do any of the yoga practices offered in this book. Why not run, hike, cycle, or walk, and then come home and do your yoga practice? Some people like to do the Energy Practice, described in Chapter 4, before they go outside to walk. It can serve as a great warm-up. It will loosen up your muscles, get your blood circulating, and deepen your breathing. Or try doing your Energy Practice after your run or hike. It will stretch your tight muscles and relax you.

Like many of our clients, you might find your own personal way of blending your activities.

Katie found that she enjoyed both lifting weights and practicing yoga. She lifted weights twice per week and practiced yoga the other five days. Some days she even doubled up her practice if she missed it on a previous day. She found that the more flexible she was, the more she got out of her weight training. She also found that her weight training increased her strength and her ability to do the standing poses and hold them longer. According to Katie, "It's all good." She has fallen so in love with movement that she added Flamenco classes to her week. To date Katie has lost 22 pounds. She has really lightened up!

Julie found that she enjoyed adding the Strength Practice (explained in Chapter 5) to the hikes she took regularly with her family. She got her cardiovascular workout on the hills, and then came home and did her Strength Practice. On other days she enjoyed the Energy Practice and the Calming Practice (described in Chapter 6). Of course, when it rained she could just practice yoga inside. This worked well for Julie's lifestyle and personal preferences. She liked being outside with nature. Sometimes she would do her practice outside at the top of a hill near her house. She told us that when she did that, she really felt like she was communing with nature as well as getting in touch with her inner goodness and spirit. What a wonderful added benefit to the 15 pounds she has lost so far!

If you're just beginning and have decided to take on the Yoga Weight Loss Program as your sole exercise, that's fine too. You will get wonderful results—losing both pounds and inches—following the programs in this book, along with the eating plan. Remember, everything is about balance. If you take on too much too soon you will not be setting yourself up for success. We want you to win!

So go ahead! Say "yes" to it all. But do it in your own time, and your own way, in a manner that is comfortable for you and doesn't overwhelm you. Yoga practice is about going at your own speed, so by all means add other activities, but do them only when and if you feel comfortable doing so. By doing your program at your own pace, you will be well on your way to health, weight loss, and self-acceptance.

Summing It Up

Hopefully now you have an overview of yoga—what it is and how it will help you lose weight. You have some sense of how to fit it into your life and you are excited about the new possibilities. Remember that the whole notion of balance is that it is a dance. There really is no such thing as a stagnant, fixed balance, but rather a gentle flux between two points that continues to become finer. Consider how you might tune in to a radio station. First you go way over to the right beyond the station and then way over the left in response. Then back and forth to the right and left in order to fine-tune the station so that it is coming in with the strongest, clearest signal.

Finding balance in our lives and in our bodies is exactly the same thing. It is not a fixed point, but a flowing state. Sometimes it will flow in one direction and sometimes it will flow in the other. If you flow (or bounce!) more to one side from time to time, don't be upset; rather, just know it is part and parcel of the journey to finding the other side and hence arriving at the balance. Finding a balance is very much a journey rather than a destination. When you slip and forget to practice, or time constraints take you away, or your kids demand your time, or you go out for a big celebration dinner and eat way more than you should, remember that it is all okay. Sure, you've disturbed your optimum balance for the moment, but you did not "blow it." You are in the balance dance. Just pick yourself up and get back on track.

Now let's move into how to set up your practice for the best results.

Chapter Three
Creating a Program That Works for You

The important thing is this: to be able at any moment to sacrifice what we are for what we could become.

—Charles DuBois (philosopher)

In this chapter we're going to talk about the kinds of things you need to do to ensure that this program will work for you. If you think about any accomplishment you've had in your life, you'll probably notice that there was some planning that went into it that stacked the deck in favor of success. For example, if you had to study for a big test, you might have made sure the phones were turned off and you had enough to eat in the house, and your family or friends knew not to disturb you. That's setting the stage for a win, and that's what we want you to do here.

Jonny often has his clients clean out their kitchens as a first step in setting up a nutritional plan. Why? Because the more obstacles that are removed, the greater the chance for success. Preparation is everything. You don't need a ton of chocolate chip cookies lurking in your kitchen cabinets just waiting for that midnight hour when your defenses are down and you feel like giving in to temptation.

In keeping with the idea of preparation and readiness, let's talk about some of the issues you might want to think about—both practical and spiritual—that could help you immensely in achieving success on the program. Let's try to answer the question: "What do you have to do to make any program work for you?"

Walking the Middle Path

One of the things that derails people when they start a weight loss program is the story they tell themselves about their possible success or failure. This can take two directions, neither of them great.

In one scenario, you tell yourself how wonderful this is all going to be, how successful you are going to be at it, how terrific the result will be, and then, if it doesn't happen exactly the way you planned it, you throw up your hands and give up.

In the other scenario, you enter into a weight loss program feeling deep down that it won't work. You believe on some level that you're going to fail again and are certain that this disappointment will speak volumes about your ability to have the kind of life you want and be the person you want to be. Sure enough, this second scenario is almost always a self-fulfilling prophecy.

We're going to suggest that you enter into the Yoga Weight Loss Program in a different way. In yoga it's called "Walking the Middle Path." It requires that you give up something—namely, your expectations. You have to rekindle your sense of wonder and your ability to be surprised. We don't expect you to fail, and we don't expect you to expect yourself to fail, but neither do we want you to have expectations of perfection. We want you to be present in the moment, and that means being with whatever is true for you. It means giving up the right to make up a "story" that defeats you either by demanding that you achieve some standard of perfection, or by expecting that you will be a failure.

Just be willing to be where you are.

Be Clear about Your Goals

Read any book that discusses the lives and careers of people who have been successful, and one thing jumps out at you: They all had definite, clearly stated goals in mind. Sometimes these goals are very big and very specific—like winning the heavyweight championship in boxing—and sometimes they represent steps along the way to a bigger goal (like losing 10 pounds on the way to 100). But setting goals is integral to success. Ask yourself how much weight you would like to lose. Don't be hung up on the number, and for goodness' sake, don't pick some unrealistic number, like what you once weighed in high school 20 or 30 years ago. What would you be comfortable with? What's a manageable weight for you to maintain after you've achieved it? What could you live with happily? Write down that goal weight and continue to monitor your progress so that you can see yourself getting there. Remember, if you know where you're headed, you're going to be much more effective at getting there. If you don't have a clear idea of the direction you want to go, you're more likely to spin your wheels in a circle and wind up in the same place you started.

We strongly suggest using the scale to monitor your progress. This may seem counterproductive to many people who have experienced the "tyranny" of the scale and have done all they could to liberate themselves from obsessing about the number of pounds they weigh. We understand completely. What we propose, however, is a more gentle way of using the scale—not as something to beat yourself up about, but as a general guide to your progress. Ideally, if you have access to a facility that can do body-fat measurements (many health clubs, for example) this would be even better than the scale because it more accurately reflects a change in body composition. (You could, for example, gain two pounds of muscle and lose a pound of fat; the scale would only reflect a one-pound difference, but in fact a much more significant difference took place in your body composition.) In the absence of body-fat measurements, don't be afraid to use the scale just as a way of "checking in."

You should be sure to use the same scale each time. Comparing results on different scales is always frustrating because any scale can be off by a couple of pounds or more. You should also weigh yourself at the same time of day (we recommend first thing in the morning); in the same state of dress (we recommend undressed); and preferably before eating or on an empty stomach. This will eliminate as many variables as possible and give you a consistent measure of your progress. We also recommend taking waist and hip measurements at the start of the program and checking these consistently at least every month.

Both of us, in our private practices and seminars, are frequently asked the question, "How long will it be before I start seeing results?" The correct and truthful answer—though not the most popular one—is "It depends."

What does it depend on? A host of factors, ranging from how consistent you are in your exercise and how careful you are with your eating to individual metabolic factors such as how easy (or hard) it is for you to lose weight. For the most part, we would say that you should expect to see measurable results within four weeks. We have certainly seen some people respond much more quickly to the kinds of changes in eating and activity discussed in this book, and we have often seen some people who respond more slowly. The point is not to be discouraged and to continue with the program, making adjustments (especially to your eating plan) as needed to support ongoing progress.

We suggest that you be willing to do the yoga program for an absolute minimum of 20 minutes a day, five times a week. We've designed it in a modular way—there are, as you will see in the following chapters, 40-minute and 20-minute versions of the workouts, and they can be combined in any way that you like. You can put two 20-minute routines together for one 40-minute routine, or do a 20-minute routine twice (or even once) a day. You can combine a 40-minute routine with a 20-minute routine. And as we discussed in Chapter 2, you can combine one of the routines with other exercise that you might already be enjoying, such as weight training, walking, jogging, hiking, or bicycling. You can certainly practice seven days a week, if that is your preference. Remember, this program is for you, and ultimately you should be the arbiter of what works best in your lifestyle. The recommendations we make are just that—recommendations, there to support you in getting results. They are not absolutes. As each practice unfolds, it will undoubtedly be as unique as the person practicing it.

Which is exactly how it is supposed to be.

Be Willing to Be Surprised

We want your yoga practice to unfold like a good story—one in which you don't know the ending and will find unexpected surprises at every turn. The fact is, you don't know the "ending" of this story. If we're successful in this book, your practice will become integrated into your life and the results will go considerably beyond the weight you'll lose; we anticipate they'll be expanding and unfolding for a very long time.

Christy Kimbro, owner of YMI Yoga Studio in Los Angeles, says she's seen it a million times: "The girls all come in here initially with their makeup and perfect hair hunting for celebs and wanting to do yoga because it's the trendy thing to do—but within a month they're completely turned around, they show up with no makeup, ponytails, and yoga mats ready to work. They really fall in love with it. They find it fills a need in their lives."

We suggest that the reason for that is simple: Yoga speaks to who you are.

See, most diet and exercise programs can be—and usually are—done unconsciously. They are like painting by numbers: You follow the food list or the exercise prescription exactly as written, no muss or fuss. Problem is, those programs are totally disconnected from who you are. Molly Fox's Yoga Weight Loss Program is different. You can't do it unconsciously. Who you are drives the program rather than the other way around. Obviously this part of the system appealed to you, or you wouldn't be reading this book. This program is about practicing the art of doing. You enter your practice in the moment. It's not about making some long-term commitment that you may wind up using later to beat yourself up when you don't stick to it exactly as planned. By stepping on the mat and trying the first pose, or by waking up and consciously asking yourself "what am I going to have for breakfast?" you're practicing the art of mindfulness, and you are "doing" yoga. You don't have to make a commitment, you just have to be in the moment. You're practicing making a choice, not being attached to the result. Your job is to apply yourself to the task at hand and not to worry about the result.

It sounds redundant, but it is true: The result will be the result. Let it unfold. Be willing to be surprised.

One part of the "who" in this equation is deciding that you need this time for yourself. Many people, particularly women, often feel that the demands of others are more compelling than their own needs, and wind up putting their own needs last, as we discussed at length in Chapter 2. You have to decide that this is for you and that you matter. Remember, if you don't take care of yourself, you can't fully be there for anyone else.

So tell your family that this is what you're going to do, and enroll them in giving you support. Explain that you need this time to practice and that it's important to you, and not to interfere with it. Get the people around you on board; they don't have to do the program with

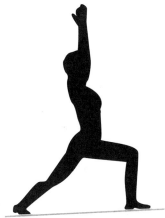

Your job is to apply yourself to the task at hand and not to worry about the result.

you, just respect and understand your desire to do it. You'll be surprised at how supportive people around you will be when you show them how serious you are about getting started on the program.

Since the program is all about mindfulness, we're going to ask you to be mindful right from the start. Plan your week. Which of the routines will you do? Will you follow the routine as stated? Will you modify it because of a busy week? Make a plan at the beginning of the week and stick with it. If you have to deviate from the plan, do it mindfully. **Choose** to deviate if you need to.

Plan Your Work and Work Your Plan

Success is a funny thing—it's all relative. And it's all dependent on the goals you set for yourself. If you go into a gym and tell yourself you're going to work out hard for an hour but you only do 20 minutes, your brain logs that as a failure. After all, you set the goal of one hour, but didn't attain it. Your brain doesn't give you "credit" for the 30 minutes; it just records "loser" in your subconscious! On the other hand, if you tell yourself you are going to do 20 minutes and wind up doing exactly that, your brain jumps for joy and registers a resounding success. The success is not necessarily in the result (the 20 minutes were the same in either case), but in the difference between what you intended and what you did. In the first case (goal: one hour; achieved: 20 minutes) there was a big difference between intention and result. In the second case (goal: 20 minutes; achieved: 20 minutes) there was perfect congruence between the two and you wind up a winner! If you take every action with mindful purposefulness, you set yourself up for success. So plan your work and work your plan.

Direction, Not Perfection

What will you eat this week? Make a grocery list. Get your family on your team. They don't have to eat the exact same way you will be eating, but they need to support you in your effort. Think of them as rooting for "Team You." Make a plan and make it happen by working it. Remember, we're not looking for perfection here, just direction.

Don't underestimate the importance of making this plan. When you take off on a plane flight, the pilot charts the course of the aircraft. But he doesn't necessarily go in a straight line. Weather conditions may demand that he fly a little to the east, to the west, higher or lower, or even land at an adjacent airport—but he never loses sight of his destination, even if he has to take an occasional detour in order to get there safely. Your life is much like that plane flight. Make your plan, but be willing to adjust to conditions—just do it mindfully. Go with the flow, but know the direction you want that flow to take. Ultimately, the flow will go with you.

Remember, even if you eat mindfully and consciously just 80 percent of the time, you're way ahead of the game and you've begun the program in a positive way.

In the journal we're going to suggest you keep to record the food you eat, it might be an excellent idea to start each week with some clearly stated intentions and goals. For example, you might ask yourself:

Which yoga routine will I do this week?

_____

_____

What changes in my eating will I make this week?

_____

Write these down and commit to them emotionally. Create a vision for what you want to achieve that week, and then get emotionally connected to it. Notice we didn't say "attached." Remember that the result will be the result. Your job is to play the game full out. Keep in mind that the greatest home-run hitters in the Baseball Hall of Fame were also the players who had the most strikeouts. But they kept getting up to bat!

When Will I Practice?

Think about it. Some people are morning folks; others don't come awake until the middle of the day. Respect your internal rhythms and work with them. This is part of planning your work (and working your plan). Which time of day will work best for you?

Remember, we're trying to set the stage for success, and that means taking into account what your life is really like. (Don't pick 7 P.M. every day if you know that you are truly exhausted at that hour.) In our experience, many people who exercise in the morning feel they are able to maintain their workouts more consistently. Exercising early in the day gives you less time to make up excuses to avoid doing it! Also, the unfolding of the day will invariably bring dozens of distractions and diversions that will feel like good "reasons" not to get to your yoga practice—that's called "resistance"! If you schedule your practice in the early part of the day you will not only "get it out of the way," but it will come to set a tone of positive energy to get you through the rest of the day. You will have begun the day by doing something good for yourself, and that will unquestionably color your mood, attitude, and energy for the rest of the day's events. Trust us on this: It always happens.

On the other hand, many people have schedules that just don't permit them to start their day with exercise, much as they might like to. And still others simply are not "morning people."

And just as there are many experts who feel it is better to exercise in the morning, there also are a number of experts (such as neurologist Dr. Phyllis Zee of Northwestern University, who spoke to CNN about this very issue in May 2003) who feel that late afternoon workouts are best. After hearing many experts voice their opinions on this matter—which, by the way, has no definitive answer—we feel strongly that the time of day you exercise is insignificant compared to the fact that you exercise consistently. It's not *when* you do it, but that you *do* it. Find the time of day that feels right to you—either for your schedule, your energy levels, or any other reasons that are unique to your life—and then just go for it. You might consider answering the following question in your journal before beginning:

What time of day will work best for me?

This is the fun part. Create your own personal yoga sanctuary. First, find a place that is yours, where you can get some privacy. If there's no permanent place like that in your house or apartment, choose a space where you won't be disturbed, and make it your own. Remember that the environment very much affects the quality and feeling of your practice.

Let your sanctuary express who you are. Some people do this with pictures, others use crystals, chimes, fresh flowers, or a waterfall. It doesn't matter. Choose things that move you. Make the space sacred—special in ways that speak to you.

Here's another question that you might want to answer in the front of your journal. You can begin thinking about it right now. Visualize your ideal place to practice, and then see how close you can come to creating it. Even if it's just a little corner of a room, you may be able to create the essential feeling of what you are looking for.

What things am I going to put in my yoga sanctuary/sacred space?

No matter where you decide to practice, make sure the floor is sturdy. A wood floor is the best, although carpet is okay as long as it is not too thick. The temperature of the room should be comfortable—certainly not too hot or too cold. (There is one school of yoga, Bikram, that practices in a very hot room, usually over 100 degrees—but that's not our aim here!)

In your sacred space you will be making every effort to limit distractions. Put your answering machine on. In fact, if you are able to, turn off the ringer on your phone. Don't have the television on, and if it is on somewhere else in the house, try to have the volume turned down enough so that it won't intrude on your thoughts or disrupt your concentration. It's perfectly fine, however, to have calming, gentle music playing on a CD player. Many CDs have been made just for the purpose of accompanying a yoga or meditation practice and listening to them may very well enhance your experience of the program. These CDs are widely available in many bookshops, particularly those that cater to spiritual topics.

What Else Do I Need?

While the following items are not absolutely essential to beginning the program, they are certainly helpful. You might want to consider getting them as soon as possible.

A Yoga Mat

The yoga mat has a kind of sticky feel to it. It is different from the typical mats that you see in health clubs, which are meant to simply provide cushioning when you lie on them and stretch or do abdominal work. The yoga mat is meant to stay put under your feet and not slide while you work on it, which is why it is thin and sticky. Yoga mats are made in different degrees of thickness, so if you like a more cushioned feel you can certainly get that without sacrificing the essential stickiness of the mat. They're available at any sporting goods or health food store.

A Strap

The strap is used in the Energy Practice (Chapter 4) for our leg stretches. It is a valuable tool for your yoga practice, and once you've used one you won't want to be without it.

Mats and straps are often available as kits in many health food stores and groceries such as Whole Foods and Wild Oats.

Why Are You Here?

People enter into a weight loss program—and a yoga practice—for very different reasons. Maybe it's to look better naked. Maybe it's to be around longer for your kids (or your grandkids). Again, it doesn't matter. Any point at which you enter is the right point. There are no "better" reasons; any reason you want to lose weight is the perfect reason, and the same goes for starting a yoga routine. You just have to be where you are.

Take a moment and jot down answers to the questions below. Your responses may help you understand yourself better, as well as contribute ultimately to a more meaningful practice. Write whatever comes to mind, and don't think about it too much. Whatever you write is what you are supposed to write. Remember, this practice is about being in the moment, fully conscious, and that means telling the truth about what's so. You can start practicing that right now!

How will losing weight change my life?

What would I do if I lost weight that I wouldn't do now?

What would the change in my body make me feel like?

How would my relationships change?

My career?

My health?

My shopping style? (What would I buy that I've been putting off?)

Remember, there's no "right" way to answer these questions. Some people visualize themselves at their target weight and imagine that the first thing they would do is run right out and buy two pairs of fabulous jeans. Others imagine going on a beach holiday where they would finally feel comfortable in a bathing suit. Still others imagine feeling more comfortable having sex (and this applies to men as well as women). Just write what's true for you.

How would I feel if I could be the person I really want to be right now?

Here are some additional tips we've found to be helpful. They may not always be possible for you to do, but they are worth considering if they are practical for your life.

- **Practice on an empty stomach.** If this isn't possible, at least make sure that the meal you eat before practicing is a light one. The best choices are white proteins (fish, turkey, chicken) and vegetables. When there is food to digest in the gastrointestinal tract the blood goes there first, rather than to the muscles (which is why your mother always told you to wait an hour after eating before going in the water!). If you start exercising, the blood will be shunted to the exercising muscles and digestion will be compromised. The obvious conclusion: When your body is not busy digesting food, it has more energy to move.

- **Water, water, water.** Water is important not only during exercise, when you are losing it through sweat, but during the rest of the day as well, especially when you are on a weight loss program such as this. Why? For one thing, a great deal of what we experience as hunger is really thirst in disguise, and when we hydrate properly we frequently notice a reduction in appetite. For another, particularly when you are losing fat, it is important to flush the by-products of fat metabolism out of the system. For a third, the more water you drink, the less likely you are to hold onto water and experience the uncomfortable, jeans-tightening bloat that so many of us are familiar with. The reason for this is that when there isn't enough water coming in, the body responds by telling the kidneys to recycle the water that is already available, and the result is water retention.

  It's perfectly fine to keep a water bottle with you at all times—you are far more likely to drink water if it is right there in front of you—and we certainly advise that you keep one within grabbing distance while you're doing your practice. Though there is no definitive research on the exact, ideal amount of water each person needs, the old recommendation of eight glasses a day seems to be a good one, though in general more is even better.

Wear comfortable clothes. You're looking for clothes you can move and bend in. If your workout clothes are too baggy and loose they will get in the way; if they're too tight, you'll feel constricted. Comfort is the key word here. We suggest sweat-pants (or shorts if you prefer) and a loosely fitting T-shirt. No shoes are necessary.

Work at your own rate. You may think you should be further along than you are, but that's just mind chatter and not very useful chatter at that. Be willing to be where you are. You will get stronger, lighter, and more mobile much more quickly than you think. One day you will surprise yourself and do more than you thought you could. But make it your meditation to honor your abilities on any given day rather than disparage them. (And by the way: Every day may be different!)

Pay attention to your breath. Your breath will tell you how you are doing. (See Chapter 8.) Think of it as your own personal inner guide. Remember that it is difficult to feel anxiety when you are breathing deeply.

Keep your props handy and be ready to use them to create more freedom in your pose and to make your pose lighter. Specifically, have the strap discussed above within reach, as well as a towel that you can sit on in some poses or put behind your neck when lying on the floor.

Close your eyes during meditative moments and feel the sensations in your body. Ask yourself, "How does it feel to move?" As you move, feel your muscles. Feel yourself standing on your bones. Become more conscious of the feelings in your body when you move. This will add greatly to the joy of movement.

Remember that yoga classes are much different from the aerobics or step classes you may have experienced or witnessed. They are extremely nonjudgmental and all-inclusive. Beginners are always welcome, and many yoga studios have classes just for complete beginners. Even if you join an "all-levels" class you will almost always be welcomed in and given some individual corrections and help, and virtually no one will look at you like you don't belong. You will frequently see people of all ages, sizes, shapes, and weights working together in the peaceful setting of a yoga class.

Consider getting a partner. Having a partner to either work with or to use as a support system is amazingly helpful in a program such as this. There are several reasons for this: One, you have someone with whom to share the ups and downs and triumphs (and occasional inevitable setbacks) of your journey. Two, you have built-in accountability; it is much harder to "stand someone up" for an exercise appointment than it is to simply not show up yourself. Jonny noticed that on his popular iVillage.com "Shape Up" challenges, many of the women were spontaneously pairing up—often with people in other states!—and checking in with each other on a regular (sometimes daily) basis to track progress, support each other in keeping their exercise and dietary agreements, and just generally be present for one another. The beauty of the Internet is that it makes it possible for you to do this with someone who isn't even in the same town as you! And if you can do it with someone who lives nearby—someone with whom you could actually exercise on a regular basis—all the better. You might want to do your yoga practice alone and meet your partner for long, brisk walks as an accompaniment to the program. It's all up to you. The possibilities are endless, and limited only by your own imagination!

Check with your health practitioner before beginning any program, including this one. This is especially true if you are over 40 and haven't exercised before, or if you have any specific illnesses or conditions that require monitoring. Chances are your health practitioner is going to say "Right on!" Yoga is good for just about anything that ails you, from lower back problems to fibromyalgia, but it's always good to get the go-ahead from a health practitioner who knows your individual situation.

One final question. Now that we've covered all of the basics, you may be having some feelings about all this. Maybe some anxiety or some anticipatory nervousness. Maybe you can't wait to get started. In any case, let's start practicing the spirit of the program right here, right now. Are you skeptical? Worried? Annoyed? Depressed? Elated? Optimistic? It's all fine.

Look at the following question, and then jot down your answer briefly, consciously, and mindfully. Remember the cornerstone of this program: Be willing to be where you are. Where you are is perfect just as it is. When you tell the truth about it to yourself, you can move on and create new possibilities.

Right now, in this moment, I am feeling . . .

_____

_____

_____

_____

Great.

Now look at that feeling, acknowledge it, and thank yourself for owning it.

Let's get started!

Part Two
Exercise and Lighten Up!

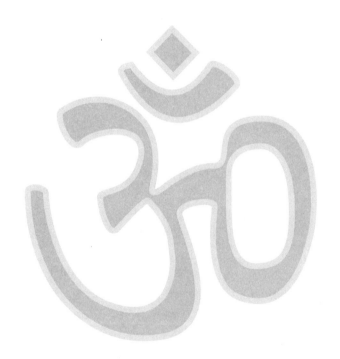

O! that this too too solid flesh would melt . . .

—William Shakespeare, *Hamlet*

Chapter Four
The Energy Practice:
40/20-Minute Versions

Every blade of grass
has its Angel that bends
over it and whispers,
Grow, Grow . . .

—The Talmud

The routines covered in this chapter will leave you feeling energized. You will burn calories and fat and you will release the hold that weight has upon you. Enjoy the process of letting go.

The idea of these sequences is to get the large muscles of the legs and hips involved and moving. Since your lower body has the most muscle in it, it is the foundation of an effective Energy Practice and is most central to both the creation of "**rooting**" energy and the burning of fat.

I have observed time and time again that my students are afraid to really use their legs. As a result, they pull energy up into their necks and shoulders—the two most common places we hold tension—and they hold their breath when moving. This restriction of the breath creates even more tension, especially in the diaphragm. You can help release this tension by being especially conscious of your legs, and letting them be involved in the poses.

Remember that there are two basic forces—with gravity and against it. When you release into gravity you allow your legs to work; they quiver, shake, and do all that other stuff that tells you they are really activated. When you release tension in the upper body, you are dropping your weight down and working with gravity. Now the deeper muscles in the lower body will start to work more. Since these are the largest muscles of the body, you will burn more calories by using them.

The bottom line: Remember to use your feet and your legs. Allow gravity to help you lose weight.

You will want to work at a moderate intensity. A moderate intensity would be one where you can use your Deep Sea Breath (described below). When you feel you have to open your mouth to get enough air in, back off a bit. Don't worry if the breath and the poses don't come together right away. Be patient—eventually they will. The most important thing is to do the practice anyway.

You will feel your heart pump, your legs shake, and your muscles burn; it's all good. Let the energy flow through your body. Think of letting go of what you are holding onto. That sensation is the universe's reminder that you are alive.

Now let's first talk about your breathing.

This is the recommended breathing practice for the asanas to follow. While it's obvious that breathing does not burn a significant number of calories by itself, breathing in this way will increase your energy and bring more oxygen to the tissues. It will make your yoga practice more enjoyable, more fluid, and more joyous. You'll be more engaged in it, you'll release tension in your diaphragm, you'll fully exercise your belly muscles, you'll feel more stable and centered, and you're more likely to experience a state of pleasure while doing the practice. You will be creating the "present moments" we talked about in Chapter 1.

If you use the breath in the recommended way while doing the asanas, you will perform them more effectively. This means you will tire less easily, you will be fully oxygenating the blood, and you will be moving the lymph fluid through the system. The result of this more effective movement is that you will get the maximum calorie burn (and other benefits) of the practices.

The Deep Sea Breath

Have you ever noticed the soothing, cooling nature of the sea? Have you put your ear to a seashell and immediately felt the calming effects of the ocean? It is amazing how powerful the image of the sea is to our well-being. We use this image to help us visualize a type of breathing known in Sanskrit as the Ujjayi breath. For the purposes of creating a sense of calm, let's refer to the Ujjayi breath as the Deep Sea Breath. We do the Deep Sea Breath here because it helps to focus our minds, gives us something to feel and hear, and is deep and effective.

Here is a step-by-step way to get the feeling:

|||| **First, breathe through your mouth.** What do you notice? Does the air go in and out very fast with very little chance of control?

|||| **Now breathe through your nose.** Notice the difference: The breath usually moves more slowly and has a squeezing effect. The nose also filters the air, making it cleaner before it enters your body.

|||| **Breathe in deeply through your nose, and exhale the sound of Ahhhhhh out of your mouth.** Good. Let the Ahhhhhh last as long as your breath. See if you can make your inhale and exhale the same length.

|||| **Now do the same thing, but close your mouth.** Do you hear it? Can you hear the sea? Think of this as your own internal stress-reducing machine. When you practice this type of breathing it will balance your nervous system and keep you more relaxed. The more relaxed you are during your practice, the more beneficial, effective, and joyous the session will be.

When we practice the Deep Sea Breath, we want to make the sound of the sea in the throat. It should feel as if you are breathing from your throat. What you are actually doing is closing off the back of the throat—that's what is making the constriction and the sound.

Energy Practice

The Energy Practice can be thought of as the perfect "entry level" practice session. There's a lot of movement in it as it flows from pose to pose using large muscle groups. The repetition of the movements will free your body up, create energy that will burn calories, and leave you feeling strong and supple. This practice is of moderate intensity for most people.

The Energy Practice is based on rhythmic movement and flowing sequences. It has been designed in both a 40-minute and a 20-minute version so that you can fit it into your life.

Obviously with the 40-minute version you'll expand and create more than the 20-minute version, but remember doing something is much better than doing nothing at all. And the 20-minute version gives you many options for combination with other routines, as you will see in Chapter 9, the Two-Week Sample Practice.

Warm Up

The warm-up gets blood and oxygen flowing into the muscles so that they are warm rather than brittle. It warms your shoulders and spine and prepares you for the activity to come. It connects you to your breathing. Though, like many people, you may feel that you can skip the warm-up and just start jumping around, I have found that the calmer you are before you start moving quickly, the more you can access your deeper muscles and the deeper you can breathe. Think of Michael Jordan: The more intensely he plays, the more you notice that his jaw is completely relaxed—you can even see his tongue. Why? Because he has mastered the art of being relaxed in the midst of movement and tension.

The warm-up gets the muscles ready for activity. Remember that muscles are a little like saltwater taffy. When they're cold they're dry, brittle, and more easily injured, but when warm they are pliable and loose. That's why stretching should always be performed after a warm-up.

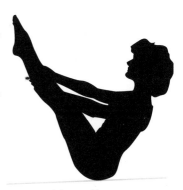

Use the 20-minute Energy Practice as a quick pick-me-up at the end of the day!

Jonny and I once studied with a great teacher who used to ask his students what they thought was the difference between a master white-water rafter and a beginner. Obviously, it is not the ability to control the water—no one can accomplish this. But the master has learned to be calm and centered in the midst of chaos. He has learned to be in control while being out of control. The breathing exercise gets us in touch with that sense of calm; it is the door to enter into what John Douillard, author of *Body, Mind and Sport,* calls the "calm in the center of the storm." It makes you enjoy your practice more. You want to always be in touch with this feeling, even while doing the most strenuous movements. That's why we begin the warm-up with 5 minutes of breathing.

The rest of the warm-up, once you are completely familiar with the movements, should take you about 5 more minutes to complete.

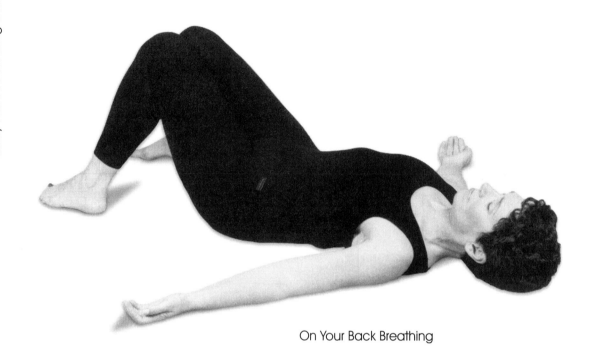

On Your Back Breathing

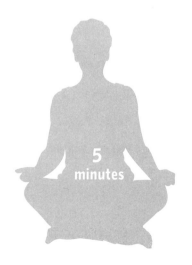

5
minutes

[On Your Back Breathing]

||||| Your knees are bent, feet flat and hip-distance apart, knees rest in and arms open.

||||| Focus on Deep Sea Breaths with an even inhale and exhale.

||||| Become more relaxed in order to access and create positive energy.

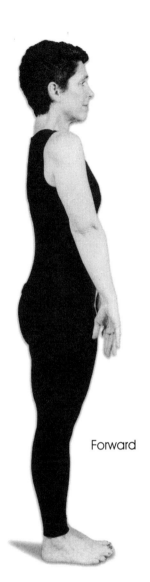

Forward

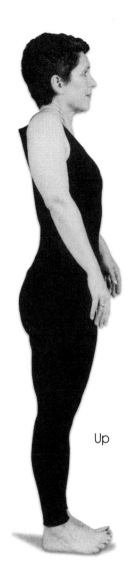

Up

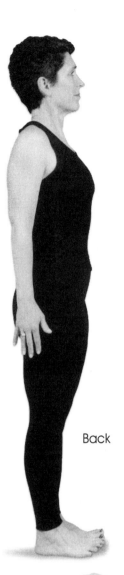

Back

[Shoulder Rolls]

▐▐▌ Roll your arm bones forward, up, and all the way back, making
the circles as big as you can.

▐▐▌ Inhale as your roll your arm bones forward and up and exhale as
your roll them back and down.

▐▐▌ Reverse rolling your arm bones back and up on the inhale and
forward and down on the exhale.

**10 rolls
each way,
sitting
or
standing**

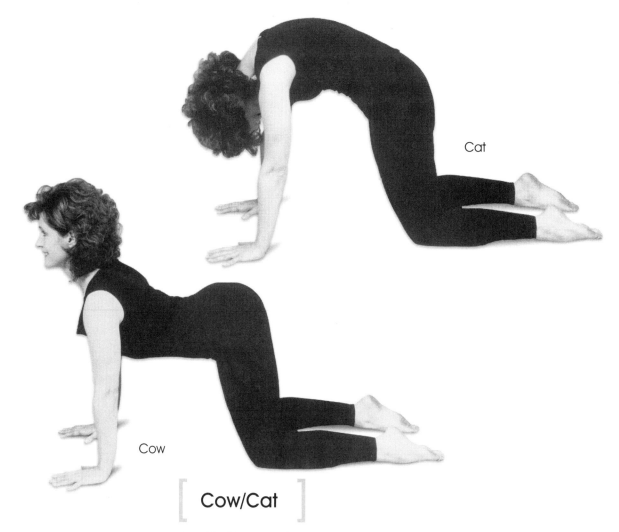

Cat

Cow

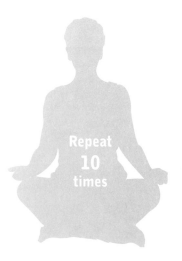

**Repeat
10
times**

[Cow/Cat]

Cow/Cat is a great way to warm up your back. You arch your back like an old cow in the pasture. (Think of the image brought forth by "the old gray mare, she ain't what she used to be.") Then you round your spine like an angry cat. That's where the name Cow/Cat comes from. It's an excellent way to warm up the spine, get the blood circulating, and to really feel how open your chest and back can be.

|||| Kneel on all fours.

|||| Inhale as you stretch your chest forward between your arms and reach your pubic bone back between your legs, letting your back drop and arch like a Cow.

|||| Exhale as you scoop your tailbone under, bringing your chin to your chest and pushing the floor away, rounding your back like an angry Cat.

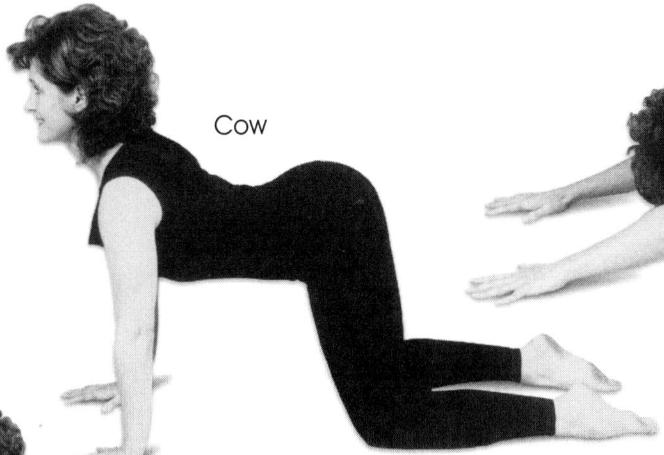

Cow

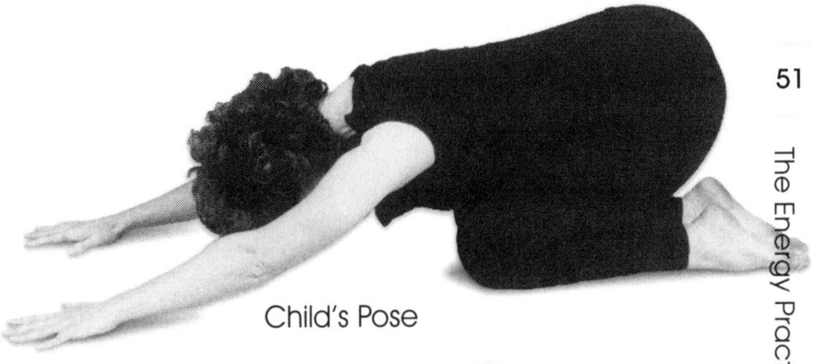

Child's Pose

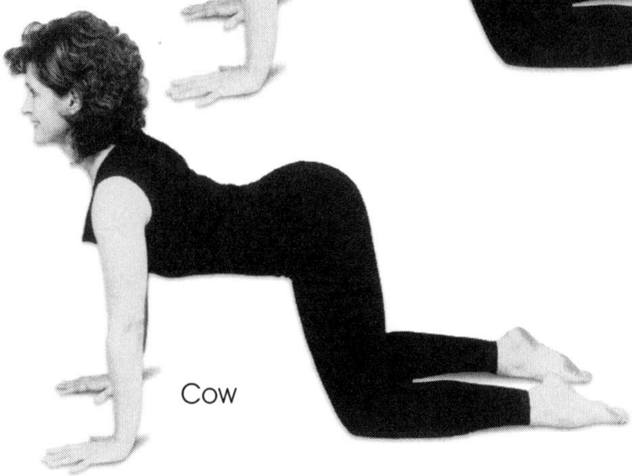

Cow

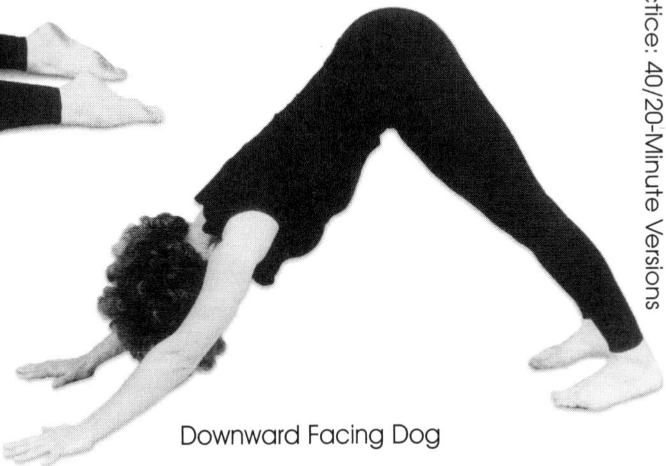

Downward Facing Dog

[Cow / Child's Pose / Cow / Downward Facing Dog]

Notice now that we're starting to move a little bit more. We're connecting our Deep Sea Breath to the movement and bringing more postures into the sequence. Don't be confused by the additional poses. Welcome them into your practice. Let the Cow Pose that you learned above flow effortlessly into the Dog Pose.

What we're doing here is linking your poses with your breathing. These poses are preparing you for the Sun Salutation below—in fact, they are a kind of "mini–Sun Salutation." Experience the fluidity of your breath together with the poses.

⦚ Inhale: Cow as before.

⦚ Exhale: Sit back on your heels, stretching your arms forward in Child's Pose.

⦚ Inhale: Cow as before.

⦚ Exhale: Curl your toes under and lift your hips up and back as you stretch your legs away from your arms to Downward Facing Dog.

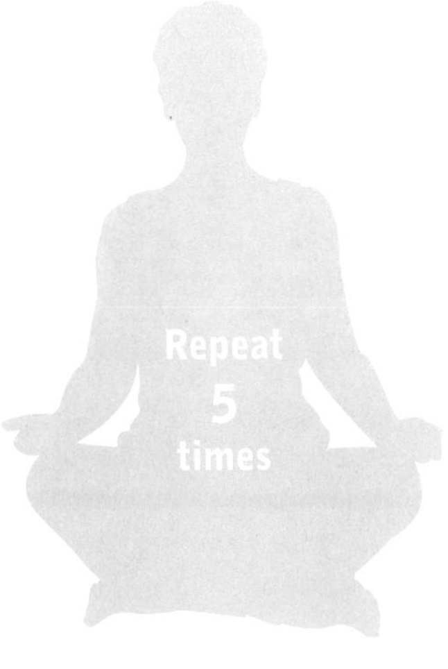

Repeat
5
times

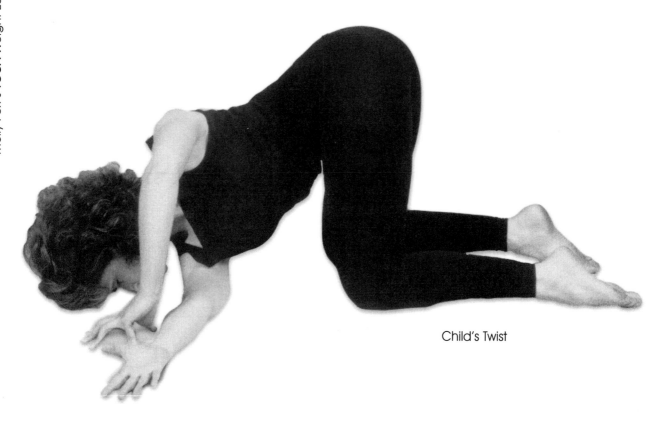

Child's Twist

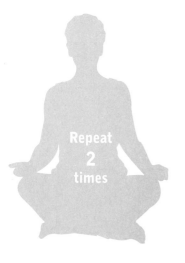

Repeat
2
times

[Child's Twist]

▐▐ From the Child's Pose (page 51) bring your hips forward so they are over your knees.

▐▐ Come onto your left fingertips, making a claw, and slide your right arm under your left so that your right shoulder is on the floor.

▐▐ Look down toward the floor.

▐▐ Hold for 5 breaths.

Sun Salutation 1 (Surya Namaskar)

The Sun Salutation 1 perfectly synchronizes movement and breath. It is the gentlest of warm-ups. We inhale as we stretch and open our chest and extend our spine; we exhale as we flex forward and close.

Your breaths in the movement should be pretty close to equal length. You can shorten your movements to match your breath until the length of your breath gets longer. Don't worry, though, if at first your breath is uneven and fragmented; it will change over time. You can even use two breaths within one movement—or take two breaths to get from one pose to the next if that feels like the best way for you. Just keep in mind the goal you are working toward: a single breath with a single movement.

Jonny used to take yoga classes in New York City where, after a while, the teacher would no longer call out the poses during the Sun Salutation, but rather simply say "inhale" and "exhale." The class would do the movements associated with those breaths because the two had become so connected in their minds.

I recommend that you start the breath a microsecond before you begin the movement, so the breath leads the movement!

I love the Sun Salutation because you really start to sweat. It's a juicy, delicious way to move your body, feel your muscles, feel your breath, and burn calories—all at the same time. When you get into the flow of it, you will see that it is really joy in motion. Many of my students will begin their day (or end it) with a Sun Salutation, even if they can't fit in any other exercise.

I find that I'm much more stable and my breath is deeper in Sun Salutation if, as I inhale, I feel like I am filling up my lower chest, then my middle chest, and then my upper chest, in that order. As I exhale I draw my navel in and secure my belly as I allow the air to go out. When I secure my belly on the exhalation it allows my chest to stay lifted and not collapse.

Stick with it, and your breath will become both deeper and freer.

Repeat 5 times

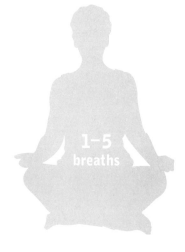

Mountain

1–5 breaths

[Mountain (Tadasana)]

From the outside, this can look like an easy pose, but if you really stand rooted on the ground with your chest lifted, your heart open, and your back drawn, you will find that it takes energy, desire, and commitment. The Mountain Pose represents the strength we get from standing up for ourselves.

When Jonny was a professional pianist, way back in the "day," he accompanied a wonderful dancer who went on to become featured in the Alvin Ailey Company and eventually to have a company of his own. His name was Milton Myers. Jonny recalls the energy that Milton used to project even when he was standing still. When he was on stage with his dancers, even when he was in the background in a stationary position, he always projected a beautiful, controlled sense of coiled energy. You never felt he was passively resting—rather, that he was supremely present in the moment, even when it "looked" like he wasn't doing anything. That energy—which you can have even when you're "standing still"—is what the Mountain Pose is all about.

Take a moment, **every time you come back to the Mountain Pose in your Sun Salutation, to** say to yourself some positive affirmation, **even if it's as simple as "You go, girl!"**

- Stand with your feet together and parallel.

- Press down through the four corners of your feet. The four corners of your feet are the inner and outer ball and the inner and outer heel. If you feel tightness in your groin, open your feet hip-distance apart.

- Firm your legs onto your leg bones and up to your pelvic core so that your hip points lift up and your tailbone scoops under.

- Firm your arm muscles so that your arm bones firm into their sockets, broadening your collarbones and bringing your shoulder blades together on your back.

- From this strong and steady stance, extend out through your feet, head, and pelvic core center like the rays of the sun.

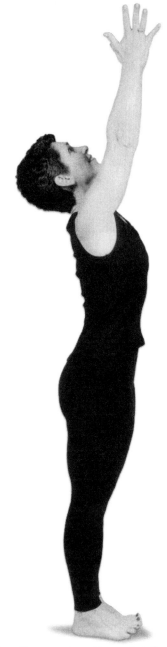

Tadasana 2

[Tadasana 2]

Tadasana 2 is about stretching the center of your body and reaching in two directions—down and up—at the same time. From the center of your belly, your legs extend down to the earth, and your chest, arms, and head extend up to the sky. This will help you achieve a long, lean look by stretching and expanding the spine, while at the same time helping to counter the effects of gravity.

▥ From a strong Mountain, inhale as you stretch your arms up, lifting your rib cage up off your pelvis and drawing your shoulder blades down your back.

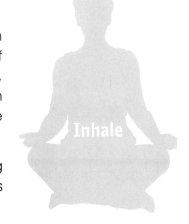

Inhale

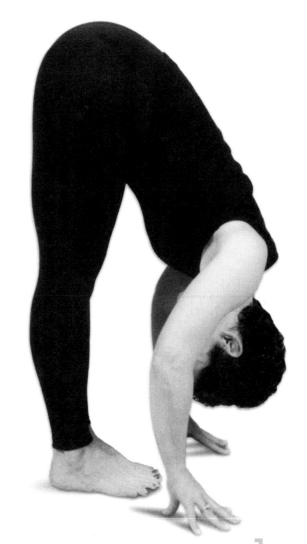

Forward Bend

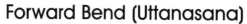

[**Forward Bend (Uttanasana)**]

The Forward Bend stretches the back of your legs—an area which is usually very tight for most of us—and allows the whole back of your body, including the spine, to stretch and expand. It also gives you a moment to "go inside" yourself; the movement itself has a quality of surrender and release. Enjoy it.

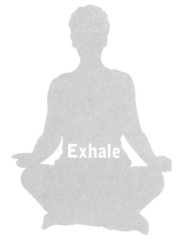

Exhale

|||| Keeping your strong Mountain, with strong legs and lifted hip points, exhale as you fold at the hips and touch the floor. Bend your knees (if necessary) to touch the floor.

|||| Stay strong in the four corners of your feet, and lift your hips up to the sky.

Intense Pose

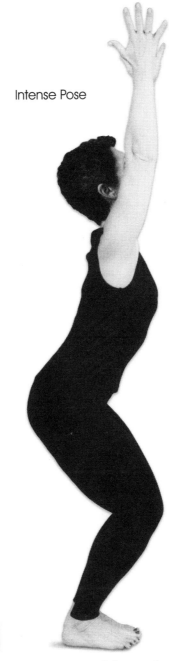

Intense Pose (Utkatasana)

Intense Pose is a fiery pose. It is alive and dynamic and uses all the major muscle groups. It generates heat and radiates vitality.

|||| From the four corners of your feet, make your legs firm.

|||| Press your heels down strongly, and bend your knees forward away from your heels directly over your second toe. This will lower your hips.

|||| Inhale. Sweep your arms up by your ears, lifting your rib cage up off your pelvis and drawing your shoulder blades down your back.

Inhale

Mountain

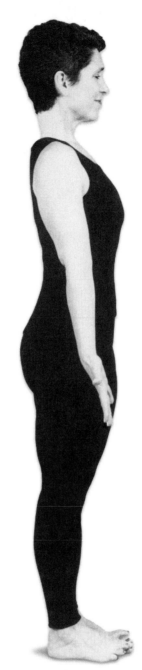

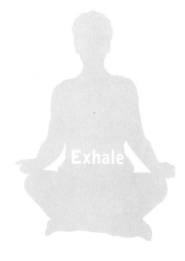

Exhale

[Mountain (Tadasana)]

We return to the Mountain Pose to complete one round of Sun Salutation 1. It allows us to get stable, centered, and reconnected to the energy of the earth. Don't forget your positive affirmation!

Exhale as you push down with your feet and back to your original Mountain. Stay strong and steady.

The goal when performing these exercises, eventually, is to move in synchronization with the breath, in a fluid and effortless manner, literally breathing through the movement. An advanced student, therefore, would be doing each movement on one breath. However that is very difficult when you are starting out. So here's what I suggest: As you are learning each pose, hold it for five breaths. That way you can concentrate solely on the movement/pose rather than on coordinating it with your breathing. As you get more comfortable and practiced, reduce the number of breaths you are holding until, ultimately, you get to do each movement on one breath, moving and breathing effortlessly.

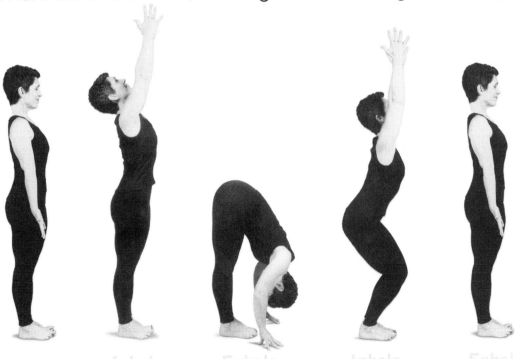

Inhale   Exhale   Inhale   Exhale

Sun Salutation 2

Sun Salutation 2 is physically more intense than Sun Salutation 1 and includes more movements. Think of it as an expansion and development of Sun Salutation 1. As you move up and down through the floor you are using the larger muscle groups, and your movements will begin to start feeling "bigger." You are now sufficiently warmed up; your heart rate is up and your breath and body are coordinated and connected. It's now time to stretch yourself a bit.

If you find that at this time that Sun Salutation 1 raises your heart rate enough and performing Sun Salutation 1 feels like exercising near your maximum comfort level, feel free to stick with it for the time being. Go ahead and do Sun Salutation 1 5 to 10 more times rather than moving on to Sun Salutation 2. When you notice you're starting to adapt to that and it gets a lot easier (or even downright boring) it's time to start adding Sun Salutation 2.

Repeat 5 times both sides

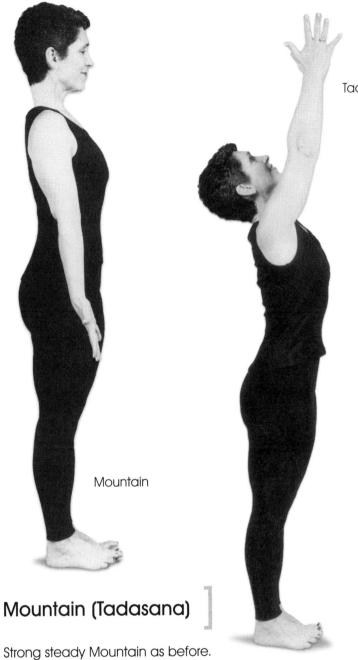

Tadasana 2

Forward Bend

Mountain

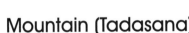

[Mountain (Tadasana)]

|||| Strong steady Mountain as before.

[Tadasana 2]

|||| From your strong Mountain position, inhale.

|||| Stretch up as before.

[Forward Bend (Uttanasana)]

|||| Keep your stretch up.

|||| Exhale.

|||| Fold over and touch the floor.

Low Lunge (right back)

High Lunge (right back)

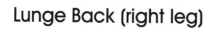

Lunge Back (right leg)

The Lunge Back is a high-energy pose and a dynamic leg strengthener. In addition to strengthening your legs, it strengthens your back and opens your chest.

▍ Inhale as you reach your right leg back to a Low Lunge.

▍ Keep your rib cage lifted, chest up.

▍ Make your back leg strong into your pelvic core so that your leg lifts up and becomes light.

▍ Keeping your pelvic core strong and hip points lifted, push down through your feet and sweep your arms up by your ears, coming into High Lunge.

▍ Make sure your front knee stays in line with your second toe and over the center of your foot.

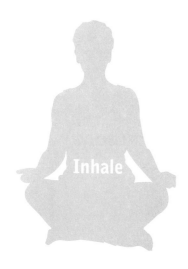

Inhale

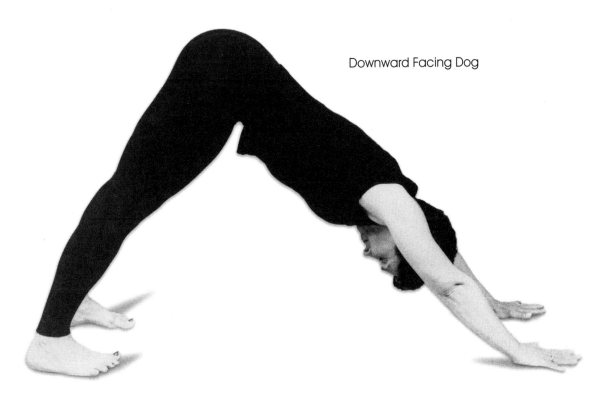

Downward Facing Dog

Downward Facing Dog (Adho Mukha Svanasana)

This pose is terrific for stretching the backs of legs (hamstrings) and for strengthening your arms while you stretch your shoulders.

- Exhale as you take your left leg back to Downward Facing Dog.

- Legs and hips extend back away from your hands.

- Muscles of your arms should be firm and lifted, which will broaden your collarbones and draw your shoulder blades back and down.

- With strong arms and extended legs, let your chest soften forward. (It should feel like you're melting your heart.)

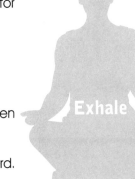

Exhale

Plank

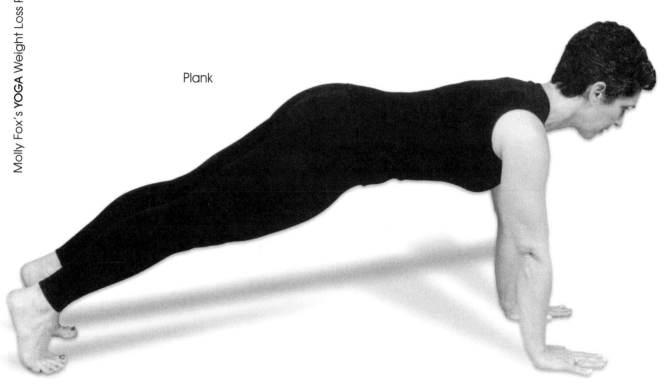

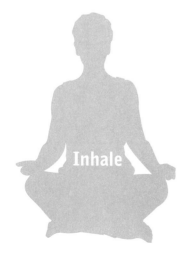

Inhale

[Plank]

This is one of the best poses of all time! It creates strength in your shoulders, your pelvis, and your abdominals as well as stability throughout your whole body.

◫ Inhale, keeping your arms and legs strong into your pelvic core, and your chest forward between your hands, bringing your body into one line—this is the Plank position.

◫ Activate your leg muscles. (It should feel like you're firing up your thighs even more than you think you are doing.) This will make your pose light and take some of the weight out of your arms.

◫ Reach your rib cage forward through your arms.

Knee, Chest, Chin
(Sun Salutation 2: Standard Version)

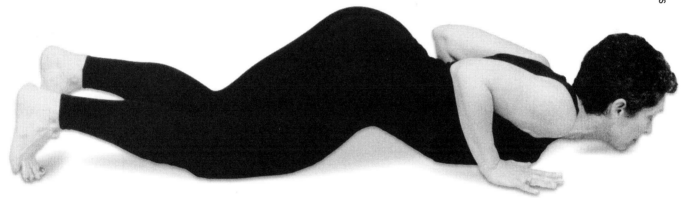

[Knee, Chest, Chin]

This is a modified yoga push-up and is great for stretching the chest and strengthening the back. It is also amazing for the development of overall coordination.

▥ Drop your knees to the floor, keeping your butt lifted.

▥ While keeping your arms super strong, shoulders back, and your chest stretching away from your strong pelvic core, exhale. At the same time, melt your heart so that your chest lowers to the floor between your hands.

▥ Look forward with your chin on the floor.

Exhale

Yoga Push-Up
(more challenging alternative)

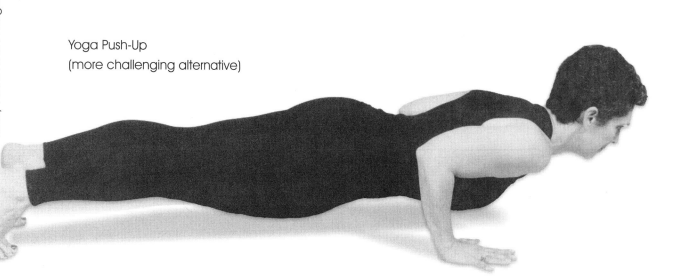

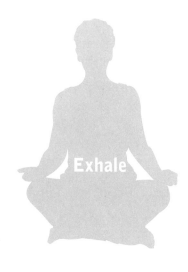

Exhale

Alternative to Knee, Chest, Chin—Yoga Push-Up
(for Sun Salutation 2: Kick-Tail Version only)

This is a more challenging option for you to do instead of Knee, Chest, Chin. Yoga Push-Up is like Plank Pose, but with your elbows bent. You come into the Yoga Push-Up from the Plank position. This more challenging option I call the "kick-tail" version of the Sun Salutation 2, because it really kicks butt!

- From Plank, press down through the balls of your feet to keep your legs strong and lifted up to your pelvic core.

- Make muscles in your arms and use that strength to keep your shoulder blades back and down while your collarbones are broad and your heart stretches forward.

- Keep a 90-degree angle at your elbow, with your elbow alongside your waist and the top of your arm bones lifted.

- Lower your strong yet light body down toward the floor.

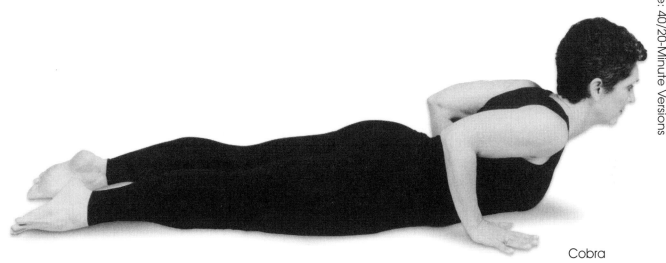

Cobra

Cobra (Bhujangasana)

Cobra Pose strengthens your back, hips, and legs while it opens your chest. Even though your legs are on the ground, remember that they are still active.

▪ Keeping your chest stretched forward, inhale.

▪ Drag your hands back as you slide your chest through your hands.

▪ Lower your pelvis to the floor into Cobra.

▪ Lift your chest, not your chin.

▪ Maintain a 90-degree angle on the inside of your elbow so that your shoulder is in line with your elbow.

Inhale

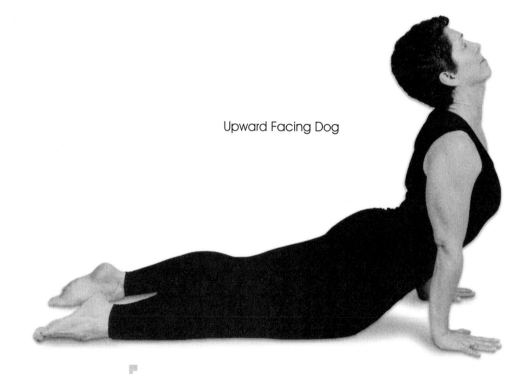

Upward Facing Dog

Alternative to Cobra—Upward Facing Dog (for Sun Salutation 2: Kick-Tail Version only)

I call this challenging pose the kick-tail version of Cobra. Since you're only balancing on your hands and the front of your feet, it strengthens your back, hips, and legs and opens your chest even more dynamically than Cobra.

If you find moving from Yoga Push-Up to Upward Facing Dog too challenging, then do the following sequence instead: from Yoga Push-Up position, lower yourself all the way to the floor, and then come up either to Cobra or Upward Facing Dog.

- From Yoga Push-Up, roll onto the front of your feet with your toes pointing backward and down. Keep your legs active and off the floor.
- Push down from your elbows to your hands to straighten your arms.
- Lift your rib cage up and forward off your pelvis as you stretch your legs back.
- From the support of your strong arms and legs, open your chest to the heavens.
- Roll back over your toes to push back to Downward Facing Dog.

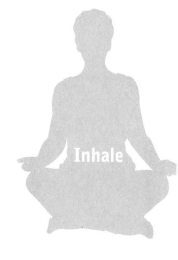

Inhale

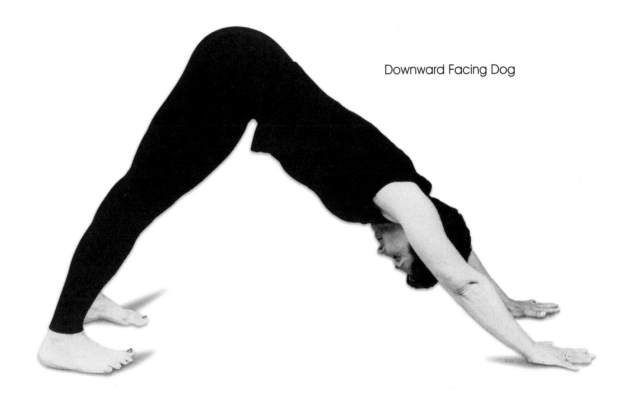

Downward Facing Dog

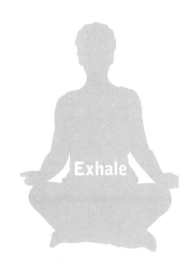

Exhale

Downward Facing Dog
(Adho Mukha Svanasana)

|||| With strong arms and lifted pelvic core, exhale.

|||| Push down with your hands to return to Downward Facing Dog.

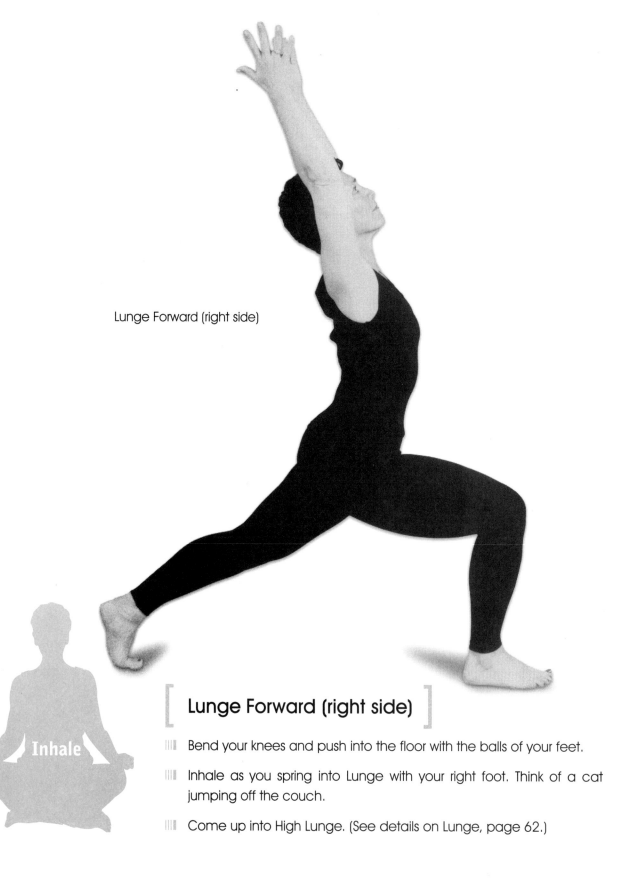

Lunge Forward (right side)

[Lunge Forward (right side)]

Inhale

||| Bend your knees and push into the floor with the balls of your feet.

||| Inhale as you spring into Lunge with your right foot. Think of a cat jumping off the couch.

||| Come up into High Lunge. (See details on Lunge, page 62.)

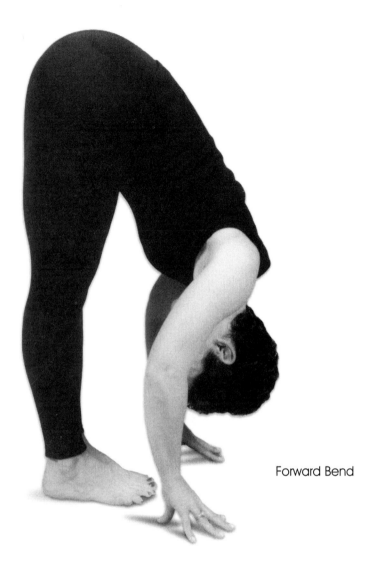

Forward Bend

[Forward Bend]

▥ Exhale as you step your back leg forward to Forward Bend, placing your fingertips on the floor.

▥ Lift your toes to activate your arches. From strong arches, lift your hip points.

Exhale

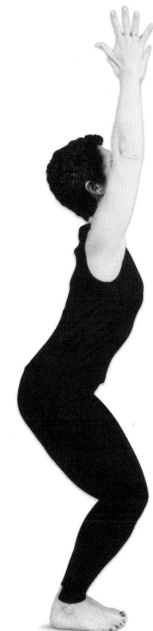

Intense Pose

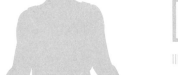

Inhale

[Intense Pose (Utkatasana)]

▥ From strong arches and hip points, press your heels down and bend your knees forward lowering your pelvis.

▥ Inhale as you sweep your arms out and up alongside your ears.

▥ Lift your rib cage up off your pelvis and press your shoulder blades down.

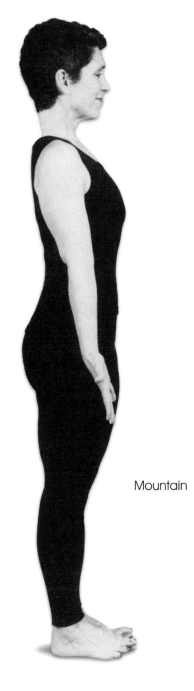

Mountain

Mountain (Tadasana)

▦ Exhale as you push down through your feet and back to strong and steady Mountain Pose.

▦ Repeat the Sun Salutation 2 sequence on the other (left) side. Then repeat the full sequence (right side and left side) 5 times.

▦ You should choose either the Sun Salutation 2: Standard Version or the Sun Salutation 2: Kick-Tail Version.

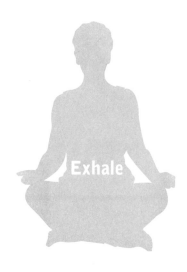

Exhale

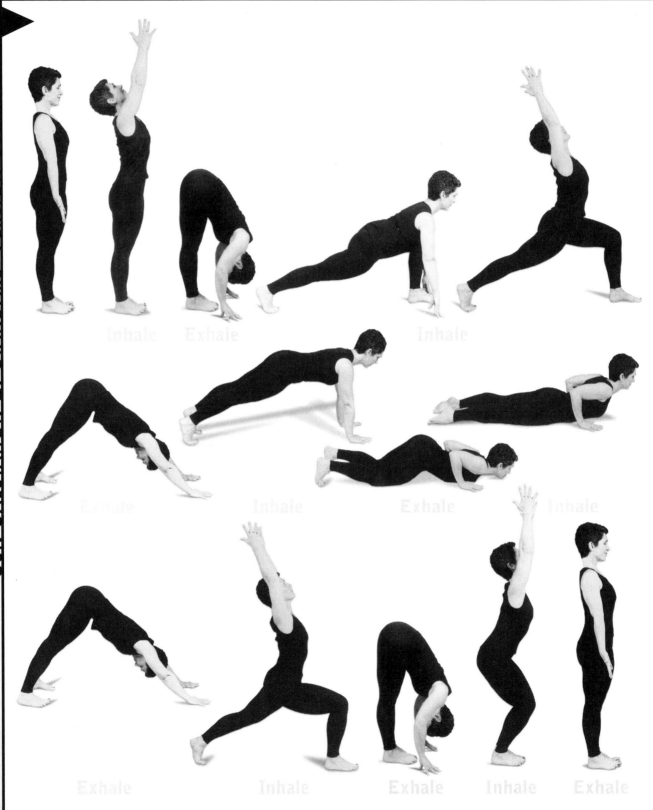

Inhale Exhale Inhale

Exhale Inhale Exhale Inhale

Exhale Inhale Exhale Inhale Exhale

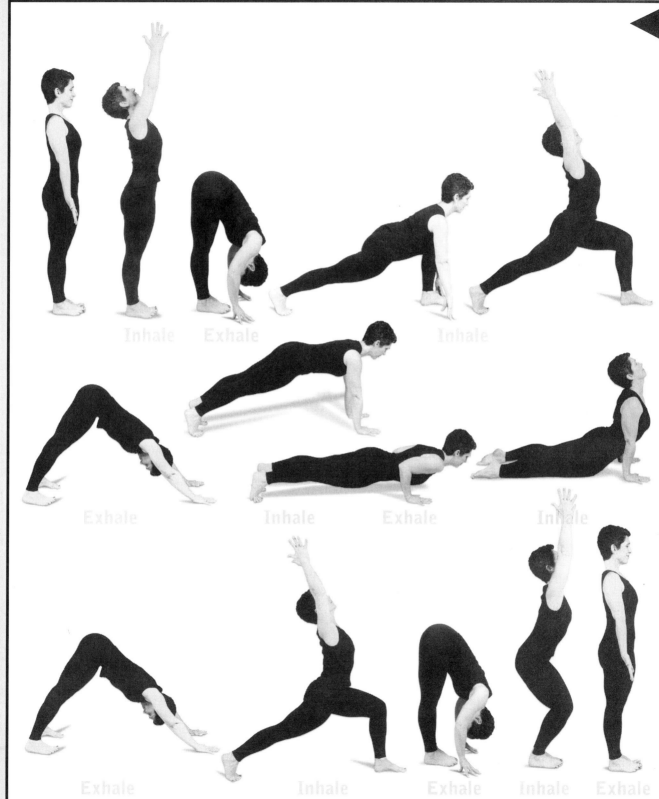

Inhale   Exhale   Inhale

Exhale   Inhale   Exhale   Inhale

Exhale   Inhale   Exhale   Inhale   Exhale

These next flowing sequences have two parts.

The first part of the sequence will be rhythmic. It will flow with your breath. We work rhythmically to slowly warm up the body and ease you into the static part coming up next. Rhythmic sequences help to loosen up stiff bodies, making your body more mobile and fluid. If you have a hard time coming into Cobra cold, for example, or if you feel stiff doing so, you'll find that this rhythmic movement will loosen you up. When you do come into the static pose, you will feel stronger and will be able to hold the pose longer.

During the second part of the sequence you will hold the pose and breathe fully. We work statically to gain more strength. Working statically will particularly benefit those people who are "looser," just as working rhythmically is of particular benefit to those who are "tighter." Working statically will increase your stability as well as your strength.

Strong Back/Open Heart Flow

This series will strengthen your back, open your chest, and strengthen your legs while you're using them to stabilize the body. Strengthening the legs (and buttocks) in this way will cause you to burn more calories and tone your lower body at the same time. Enjoy the feeling of your back holding you up while your heart stays open.

Open Heart

When we talk of "open heart" it's a kind of metaphor for a balance of effort and grace. Having an "open heart" is the opposite of being restricted. It's allowing yourself to be emotionally and physically available to your yoga practice. It's about being sturdy and firm, yet present, open, and vulnerable.

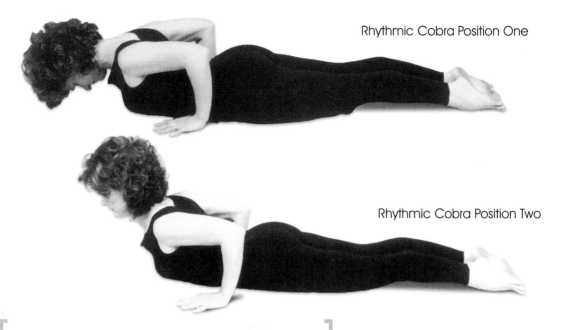

Rhythmic Cobra Position One

Rhythmic Cobra Position Two

[Rhythmic Cobra (Bhujangasana)]

This is an amazing back strengthener, and will prepare you for the Cobra Hold that comes next. The rhythmic portion of this sequence deeply strengthens both the back muscles and the top of your buttocks, creating a strong and lifted back and countering the effects of gravity on the butt that we all know too well!

Rhythmic Cobra is one of my very favorite sequences because it strengthens and shapes that very hard-to-get-at area, the top of your buttocks!

- Lie on your belly with your legs straight and together. Stretch the front of your feet long on the floor. Try to reach your fourth and fifth toe onto the floor to bring your legs more parallel.
- Move your hands back underneath your elbows and raise the top of your arm bones up in line with your elbows.
- Push down through your hands lightly and root your tailbone, legs, and feet to the floor.
- Inhale as you lift your chest and head up using your back muscles (Position Two).
- Exhale as you lower your chest down to beginning position (Position One), maintaining strong arms with your shoulders back.

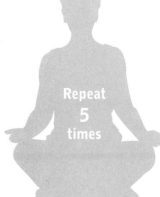

Repeat
5
times

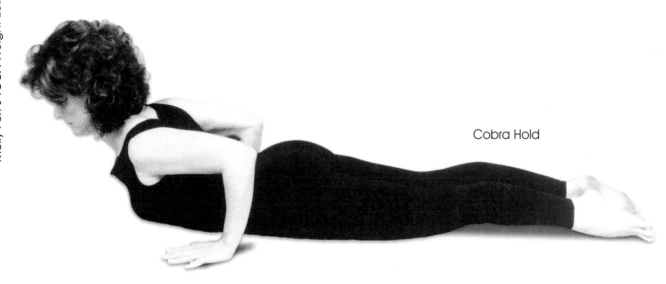

Cobra Hold

Cobra Hold (Bhujangasana)

The kind of muscular contraction you make during a hold position is called isometric—and it means contracting (or tightening) your muscles fully without motion. Think of pushing with all your might against a wall.

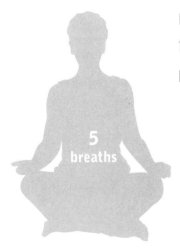

5 breaths

After doing the rhythmic kind of motion in the previous sequence, now you have to work the muscles in a different way, by holding the position instead of moving through it. It may well feel like your muscles are on fire!

|||| Hold strong yet let your breath be free. Cobra for 5 full deep breaths.

|||| Scoop your tailbone deeply into your buttocks, press your legs in and down, and stretch your chest forward, feeling your back hold you up.

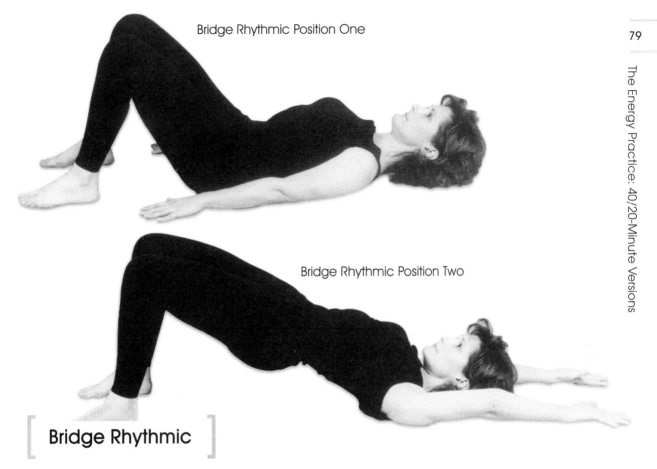

Bridge Rhythmic Position One

Bridge Rhythmic Position Two

[Bridge Rhythmic]

This rhythmic section strengthens your legs, hips, and back. Remember to press into your feet to lift your hips.

- Lie on your back with your knees bent, feet on the floor and hip-distance apart. Arms are alongside your body on the floor (Position One).

- Slide your feet back as close as you can to your pelvis.

- Move the back of your head into the floor and gaze straight up, as if you are looking straight into the heavens. This will maintain the natural curve of your neck.

- Inhale as you push down with your feet, raising your hips and bringing your arms up over your head (Position Two). By pushing down through your feet, you will feel that you're working the back of your legs instead of squeezing your buttocks to raise your pelvis.

- In this position, draw your shoulder blades together on your back and bring them down.

- Exhale as you lower your pelvis back down and return your arms alongside your hips (Position One).

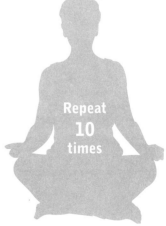

Repeat
10
times

Bridge Hold

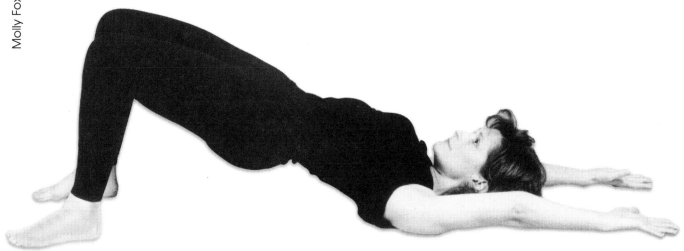

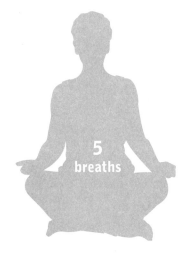

5 breaths

[Bridge Hold]

Once again, this is a static pose that will strengthen your muscles—particularly the back, legs, and hips—as you hold it.

|||| Maintaining the inhale position with your hips up off the floor, breathe deeply and fully for 5 breaths.

|||| Lower your pelvis back down to the floor.

Leg Stretch Flow

In this flow series you will stretch your hamstrings and your lower back, while at the same time experiencing a feeling of space in your hip joints. This will create more stability and freedom in your back, as well as ease of movement.

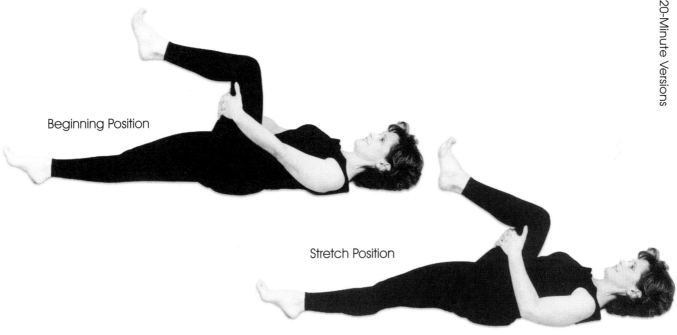

Beginning Position

Stretch Position

Single Leg Release (left and right)

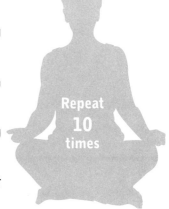

Repeat
10
times

|||| Lie on your back with your knees bent and feet flat on the floor.

|||| Draw your left leg into your chest and hold onto the back of your leg with both hands (Beginning Position).

|||| Inhale and lightly press your left leg into your hands. (This may seem counterintuitive.)

|||| Keep your leg pressing into your hand lightly. Exhale as you draw your leg in toward your chest while keeping your pelvis stable (Stretch Position).

|||| Inhale as you bring your left leg back to the original position. Repeat 10 times, followed by 10 repetitions with the right leg.

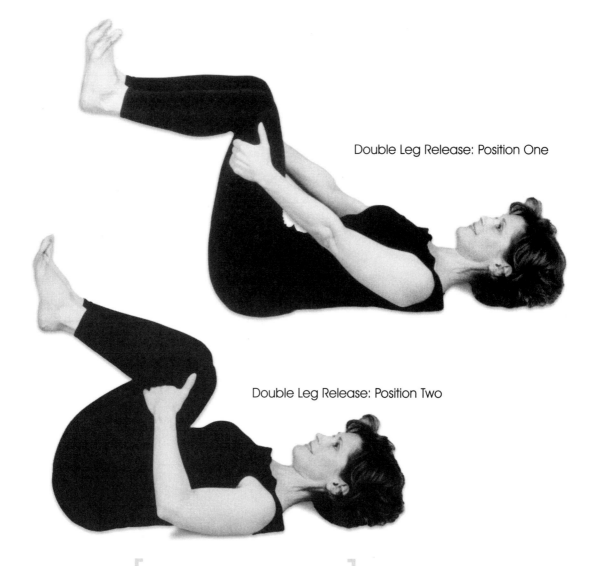

Double Leg Release: Position One

Double Leg Release: Position Two

[Double Leg Release]

||| Lying on your back, draw both knees into your chest holding onto the backs of your legs with both hands.

||| Inhale and lightly press both legs into your hands first (Position One).

||| Keep both legs pressed into your hands lightly and exhale as you draw your legs in toward your chest while keeping your pelvis stable (Position Two).

||| Inhale as you bring your legs back to the original position.

||| Since both legs will be off the floor, pull your belly in more as you exhale.

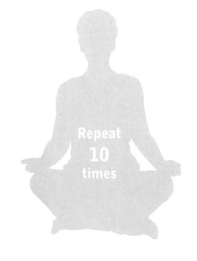

Repeat
10
times

Single Straight Leg Stretch Hold

Single Straight Leg Stretch Hold

This is a great hamstring stretch: it stretches the back of your legs and your hips. It feels fabulous, especially after you've warmed up and released your lower back in the Single and Double Leg Releases.

▥ With knees bent and both feet flat on the floor, bring your right knee in and then straighten the right leg so it is pointing straight up, and straighten the left leg so it is straight out on the ground resting against the floor.

▥ Keep your pelvis flat and assist your leg with a belt, towel, rope, or even a robe tie.

▥ Breathe deeply and fully.

▥ Repeat using the other leg.

10
breaths

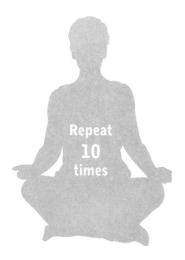

Twist Flow Sequence

This flow sequence will stretch your back and open your chest, creating more energy as you move through your day. Twisting stimulates your internal organs and will tone your abdominal muscles.

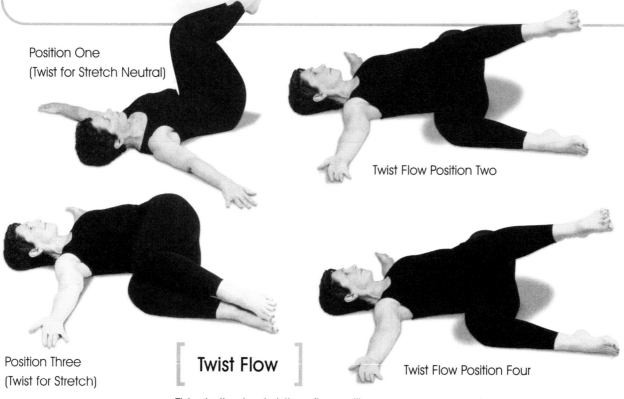

Position One
(Twist for Stretch Neutral)

Twist Flow Position Two

Position Three
(Twist for Stretch)

Twist Flow Position Four

[Twist Flow]

This rhythmic, twisting flow will warm up your spine and abdominals, preparing you for the Twist Hold. Moving rhythmically will make the holding much more enjoyable and delicious!

▥ Lie on your back with your arms out to the sides and your knees into your chest.

▥ In that position, inhale (Position One).

▥ Exhale as you lower your right leg (Position Two), and then your left, to the right side (Position Three).

▥ Inhale as you bring your left leg (top leg) up (Position Four), then your right leg back to Position Five.

Repeat 10 times

(Twist Flow continues on the next page)

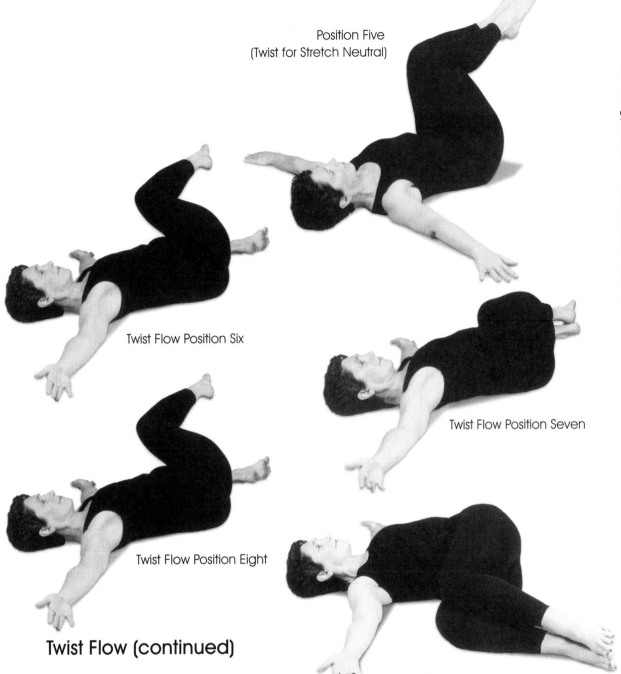

Position Five
(Twist for Stretch Neutral)

Twist Flow Position Six

Twist Flow Position Seven

Twist Flow Position Eight

Twist Flow Position Nine

Twist Flow (continued)

||| Exhale as you lower your left leg (Position Six), and then your right leg, to the left side (Position Seven).

||| Inhale as you bring your right leg (top leg) up (Position Eight), and then your left leg back to Position Nine.

||| Repeat entire sequence (alternating right and left sides) 10 times.

Twist Hold

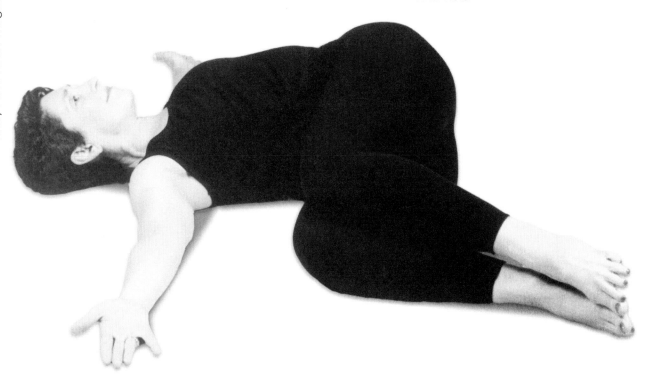

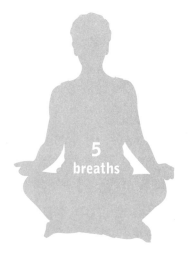

5
breaths

[Twist Hold]

After the rhythmic flowing sequence of Twist Flow has loosened up your back, you will be able to do this holding stretch with ease. You will notice a real increase in flexibility over time, and it will feel great.

▥ On your last repetition to the right, hold for 5 full deep breaths.

▥ Inhale as you raise your left leg and then your right leg to center; exhale as you lower both legs to the left and hold for 5 deep full breaths.

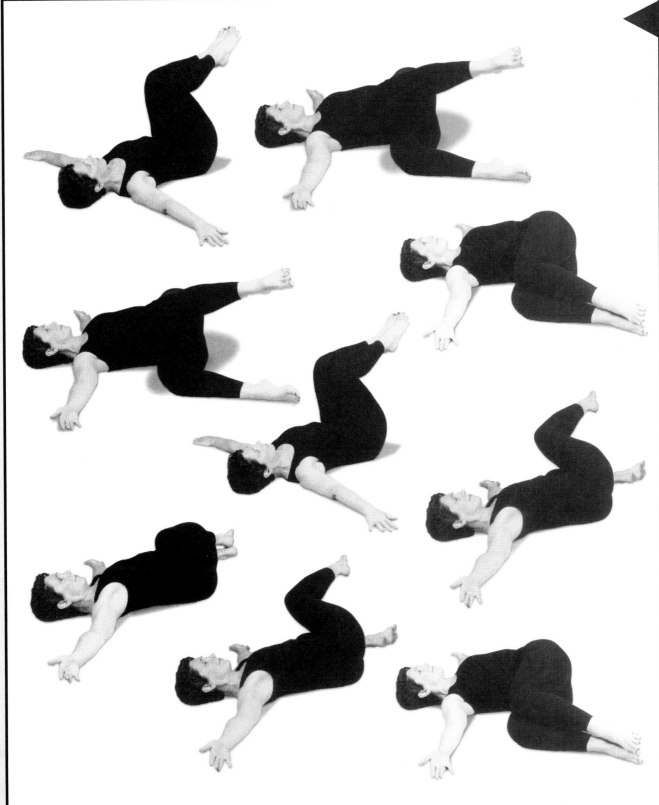

Butterfly Flow (Supta Baddha Konasana)

This flowing sequence will release tightness in your hips and create more freedom and ease of movement. It also will strengthen your inner thighs—a problem area for most women!

The more freedom you have in your hips, the more your daily movement will start to feel pleasurable and effortless; the more pleasure you feel in movement, the more activity you engage in and the more weight you lose, without even thinking about it!

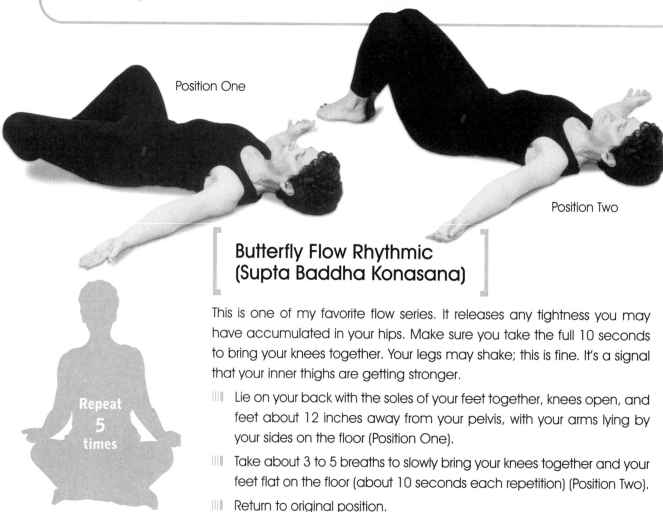

Position One

Position Two

Butterfly Flow Rhythmic (Supta Baddha Konasana)

This is one of my favorite flow series. It releases any tightness you may have accumulated in your hips. Make sure you take the full 10 seconds to bring your knees together. Your legs may shake; this is fine. It's a signal that your inner thighs are getting stronger.

Repeat
5
times

▥ Lie on your back with the soles of your feet together, knees open, and feet about 12 inches away from your pelvis, with your arms lying by your sides on the floor (Position One).

▥ Take about 3 to 5 breaths to slowly bring your knees together and your feet flat on the floor (about 10 seconds each repetition) (Position Two).

▥ Return to original position.

Hold Position Butterfly Flow

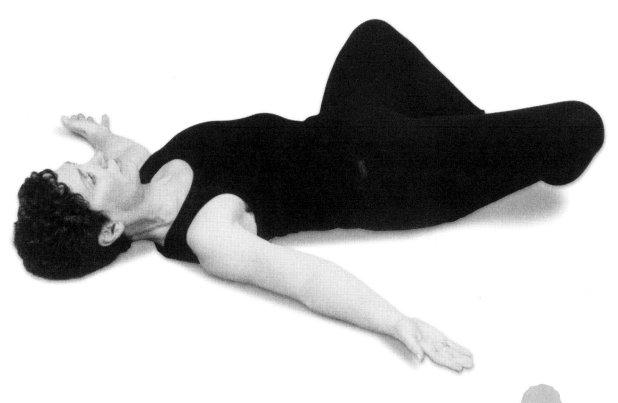

Butterfly Flow Hold
(Supta Baddha Konasana)

On your last return, hold with your legs open for 5 deep full breaths. Experience the freedom in your hips.

5
breaths

Corpse

Corpse (Savasana)

This is the deep relaxation that finally occurs at the end of the session when you finally get a chance to let all of the hard work you've done integrate into your body. You can take a deep rest. It is really a time of rejuvenation.

Sometimes people—especially driven, hard-working type A personalities—think that the Corpse Pose is a "waste of time." It's anything but. Corpse Pose is often considered to be the hardest pose of all. Why? Because it is so difficult for us to allow ourselves to fully relax. Remember, you're not trying to go to sleep; you're trying to stay conscious and deeply relaxed at the same time. If you do fall asleep, don't worry—you're probably extremely tired and need the rest. But by practicing the Corpse Pose at the end of your session, you'll be able to develop the ability to be focused and yet relaxed at the same time, giving you an incredible edge in everything from exercise to athletics to business to relationships.

- Lie on your back and allow your legs and arms to roll open.
- Cover yourself with a blanket in case you get cold. Consider setting a timer for a minimum of 5 minutes.
- If your chin is elevated higher than your forehead, place a towel under your head to make it even.
- Allow your bones to sink into the floor. Let your muscles relax off the bones, and release any conscious breathing. Let your breath breathe you.
- Enjoy the deep relaxation and the time you are taking for yourself.
- When you come out of this pose, roll to the right side into the fetal position, and then press up using the strength of your arms.

  Namaste: The divine essence in me honors the divine essence in you.

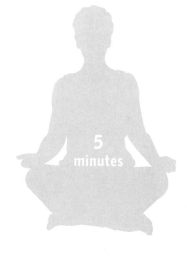

5
minutes

20-Minute Version

This is a shorter version of the 40-Minute Energy Practice. Feel free to pop this into your day when you don't have time for the longer practice, or when you need an "energy burst." I like to do this in the afternoon instead of a cup of coffee!

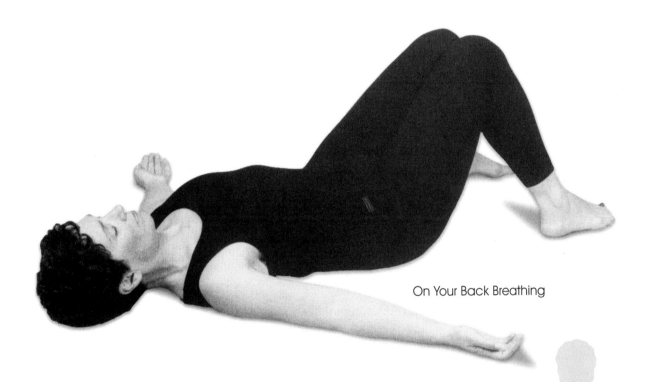

On Your Back Breathing

[On Your Back Breathing]

▥ Your knees are bent, feet flat, and hip-distance apart; knees rest in and arms are open.

▥ Focus on Deep Sea Breaths with an even inhale and exhale.

▥ Become more relaxed in order to access and create positive energy.

5
minutes

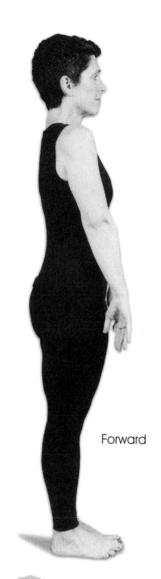

Forward

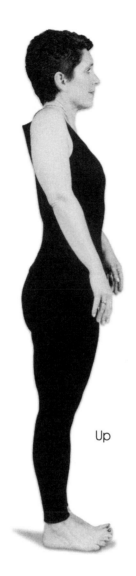

Up

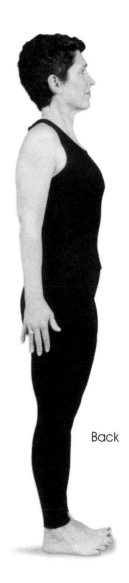

Back

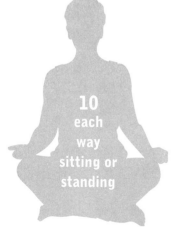

**10
each
way
sitting or
standing**

[Shoulder Rolls]

|||| Roll your arm bones forward, up, and all the way back, making the circles as big as you can.

|||| Inhale as you roll your arm bones forward and up, and exhale as you roll them back and down.

|||| Reverse, rolling your arm bones back and up on the inhale and forward and down on the exhale.

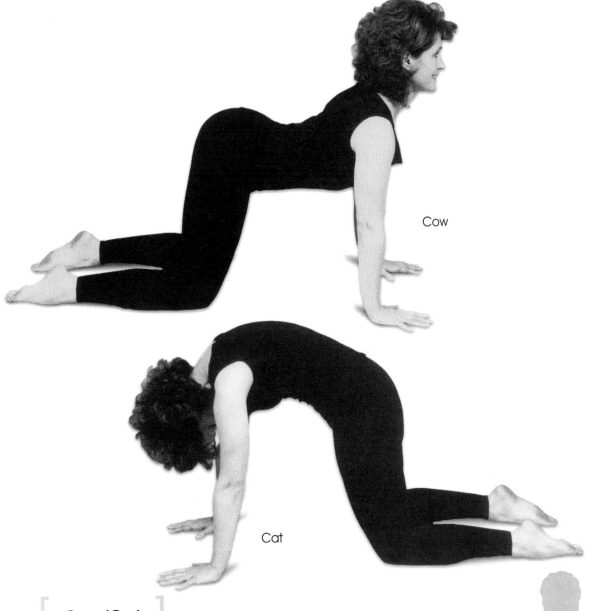

Cow

Cat

[Cow/Cat]

▥ Kneel on all fours.

▥ Inhale as you stretch your chest forward between your arms and reach your pubic bone back between your legs, letting your back drop and arch like a Cow.

▥ Exhale as you scoop your tailbone under, bringing your chin to your chest and pushing the floor away, rounding your back like an angry Cat.

Repeat
10
times

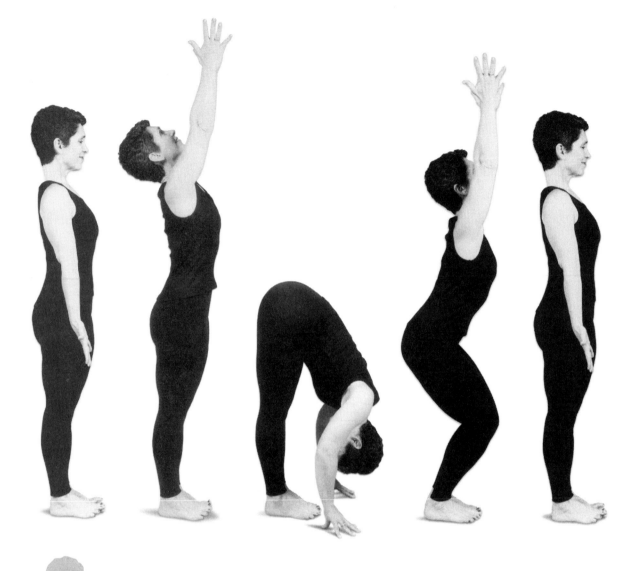

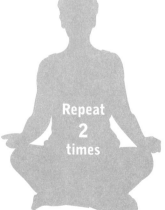

Repeat
2
times

[Sun Salutation 1 (Surya Namaskar)]

You should choose either the Sun Salutation 2: Standard Version or the
Sun Salutation 2: Kick-Tail Version.

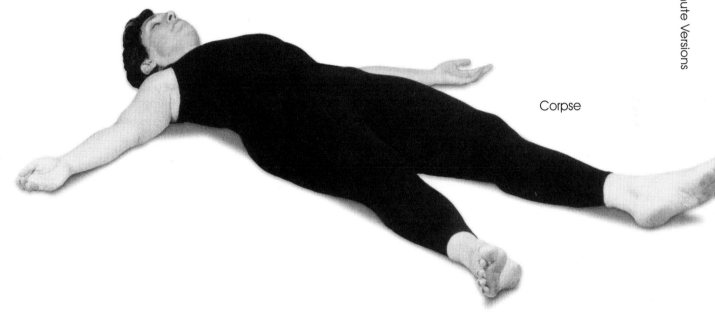

Corpse

[Corpse]

This is your time to relax and let go. This pose is sometimes the hardest, most challenging pose to do. Just be still. Bring your attention to your breath and your mind will quiet down. By committing to this 5 minutes of relaxation your day will be infused with positive energy.

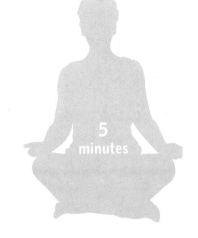

5 minutes

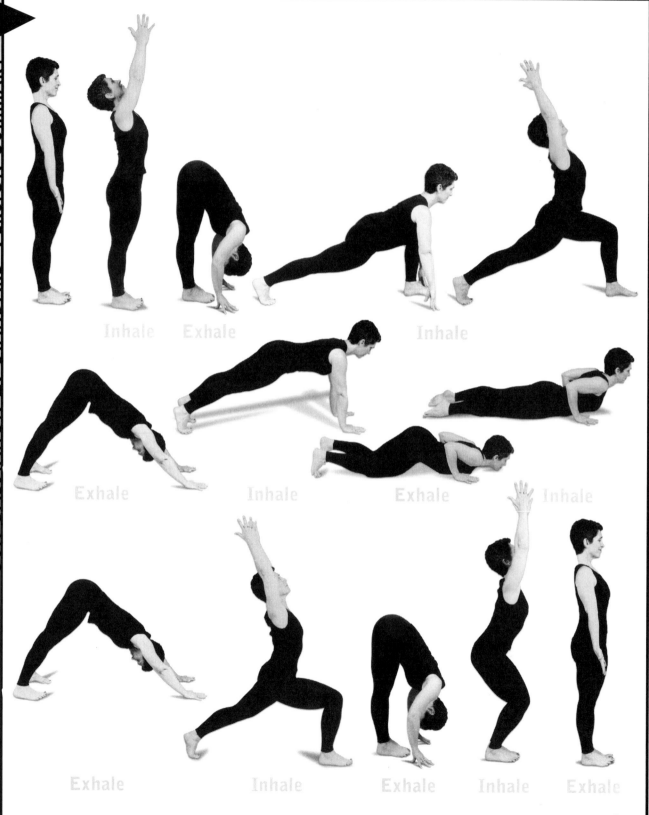

Inhale   Exhale   Inhale

Exhale   Inhale   Exhale   Inhale

Exhale   Inhale   Exhale   Inhale   Exhale

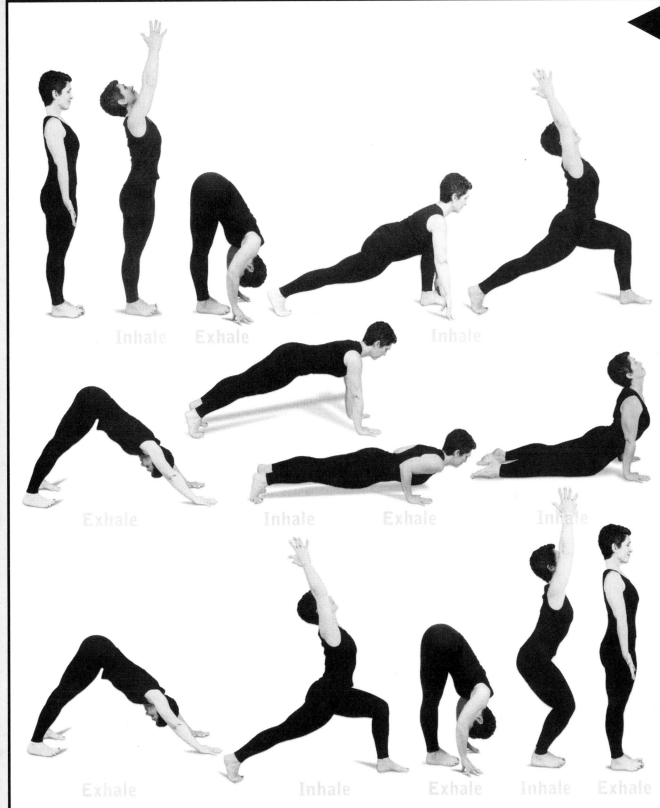

Inhale Exhale

Exhale Inhale

Exhale Inhale Exhale Inhale

Inhale

Exhale Inhale Exhale Inhale Exhale

Energy Practice Summary

The Energy Practice is a terrific energizer. You'll feel better, have more energy, and become stronger and more flexible. For maximum benefit, you should do the Energy Practice three times a week.

If you need to increase the intensity of the workout, simply increase the number of sequences of Sun Salutation 2 in any given workout or hold each position for a number of breaths. In Sun Salutation 2 you can also add repetitions—for example, repeat the Yoga Push-Up (either standard or on your knees) anywhere from 2 to 10 times. Adding repetitions of the Push-Up will increase your upper body strength, tone your arms, and of course contribute to your weight loss goals.

Don't feel that you have to master the Energy Practice before continuing on to work on the Strength Practice in the following chapter. You can use all the practices together, even at the beginner level. Your form will improve as you get more familiar with the poses. You may find that you are making more progress with one practice rather than another; this is very common and isn't cause for concern. Just allow yourself to make the progress that your body wants to make, as it wants to make it. It will all turn out well in the end.

In the next chapter we'll move on to a practice that emphasizes strength and muscle tone, increasing your metabolism for even more dramatic weight loss and fat-burning ability.

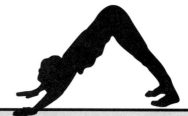

Chapter Five
The Strength Practice:
40/20-Minute Versions

Don't ask for a light
load, but rather for
a strong back.

—Unknown

The Strength Practice uses yoga poses to develop strong muscles, physical endurance, and a mental and emotional steadfastness. In this practice you will be holding your poses longer. You may need to build up to the prescribed amount of holding time, but have faith—you will develop the strength to hold these poses.

Before you begin this practice, become familiar with the poses. Practice them in advance of when you do them in sequence. That way you won't have lag time, and won't be as likely to change your mind and find yourself doing something else! It may help you to think of all the times in your life when you have been strong and successful and powerful. Bring that attitude into your practice.

Remember the quote from Henry Ford: "Whether you think you can or think you can't—you are right."

Your breathing should be natural and free. Notice whether you are holding your breath. This is just a habit, and can be changed with practice.

Breathe easy during the hard work. This practice is an intense workout for most people.

The Strength Practice

The strength practice is a dynamic yoga flow sequence that will make you strong and stable. Your muscles will become more toned, and the additional muscle will enable you to burn calories (and lose fat) more effectively, all through the day and night. As you get stronger, you'll begin to notice how much lighter you become and feel. I always feel that the stronger I get, the lighter I feel, and the more I feel a "spring in my step." Though it might seem paradoxical, it is really not. Greater strength allows you to move through the world with greater freedom and confidence, and the increased muscle mass allows you to perform and move through everyday tasks with far more ease than ever before.

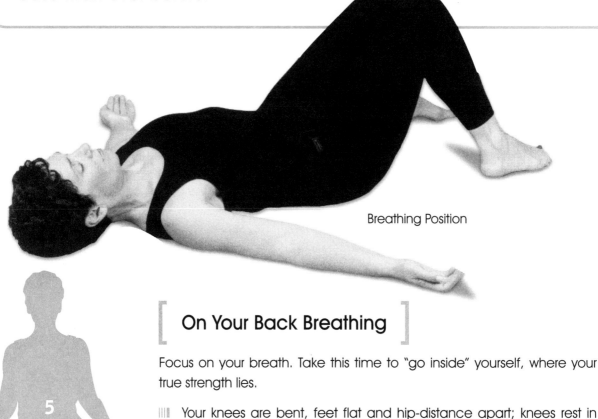

Breathing Position

[On Your Back Breathing]

Focus on your breath. Take this time to "go inside" yourself, where your true strength lies.

5 minutes

|||| Your knees are bent, feet flat and hip-distance apart; knees rest in and arms open.

|||| Focus on deep diaphragm breaths with an even inhale and exhale.

|||| Become more relaxed in order to access and create positive energy.

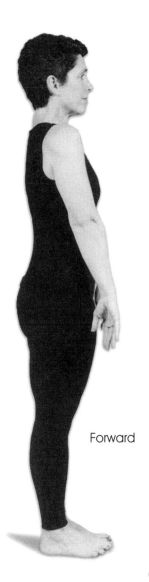
Forward

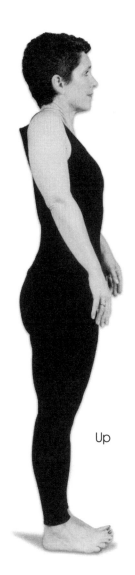
Up

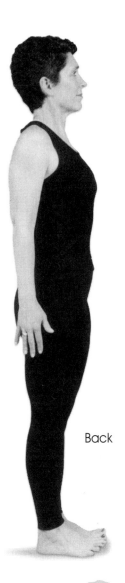
Back

[Shoulder Rolls]

Shoulder rolls warm up your shoulder joints and prepare you for the exercises to follow.

- Roll your arm bones forward, up, and all the way back, making the circles as big as you can.

- Inhale as you roll your arm bones forward and up, and exhale as your roll them back and down.

- Reverse, rolling your arm bones back and up on the inhale and forward and down on the exhale.

Repeat
10 times
forward,
10 times
back

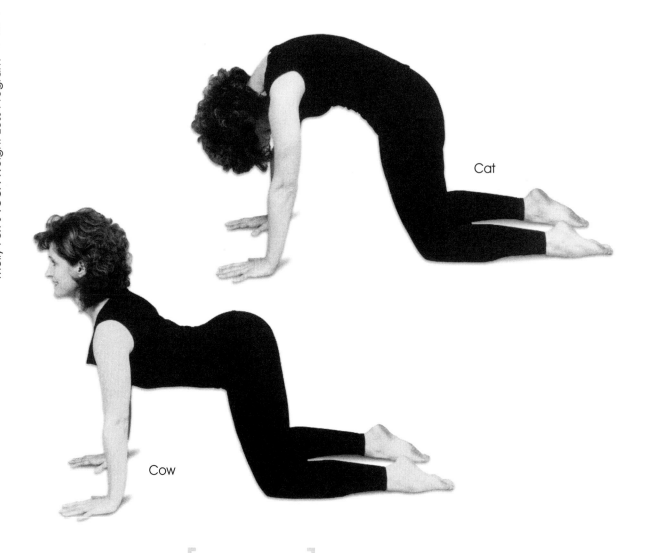

Cat

Cow

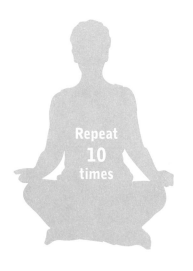

**Repeat
10
times**

[Cow/Cat]

Cow/Cat warms up your entire torso; it stretches both the back and the front of your body.

|||| Kneel on all fours.

|||| Inhale as you stretch your chest forward between your arms and reach your pubic bone back between your legs, letting your back drop and arch like a Cow.

|||| Exhale as you scoop your tailbone under, bringing your chin to your chest and pushing the floor away, rounding your back like an angry Cat.

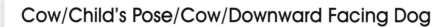

Cow

Child's Pose

Cow

Downward Facing Dog

Cow/Child's Pose/Cow/Downward Facing Dog

This flow sequence continues to warm up your back and chest as well as the back of your legs.

▥ Inhale: Cow as before.

▥ Exhale: Sit back on your heels, stretching your arms forward in Child's Pose.

▥ Inhale: Cow as before.

▥ Exhale: Curl your toes under and lift your hips up and back as you stretch your legs away from your arms to Downward Facing Dog.

Repeat
10
times

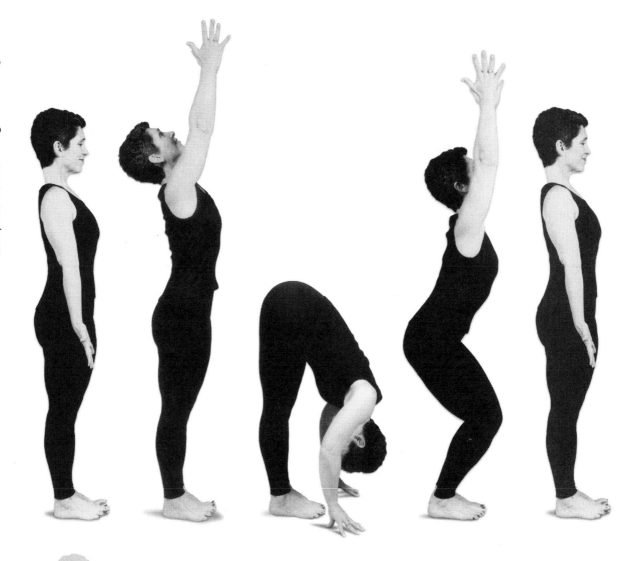

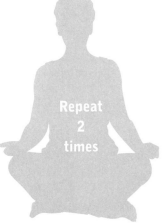

Repeat
2
times

[Sun Salutation 1]

Sun Salutation 1 will get your blood pumping and your energy flowing.
There's no better way to warm up the body! See the Energy Practice
(Chapter 4) for instructions.

Repeat 2 times

[Sun Salutation 2: Standard Version]

Sun Salutation 2 will start getting you really moving and prepare your whole body for the dynamic strength work to follow. See the Energy Practice (Chapter 4) for instructions.

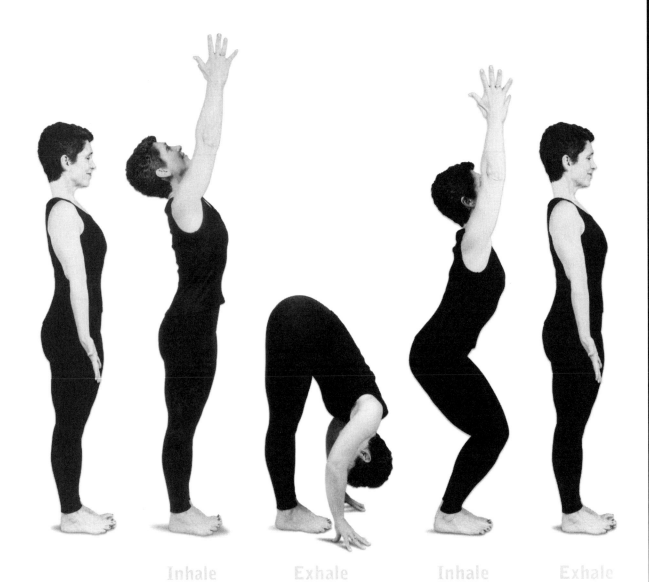

Inhale   Exhale   Inhale   Exhale

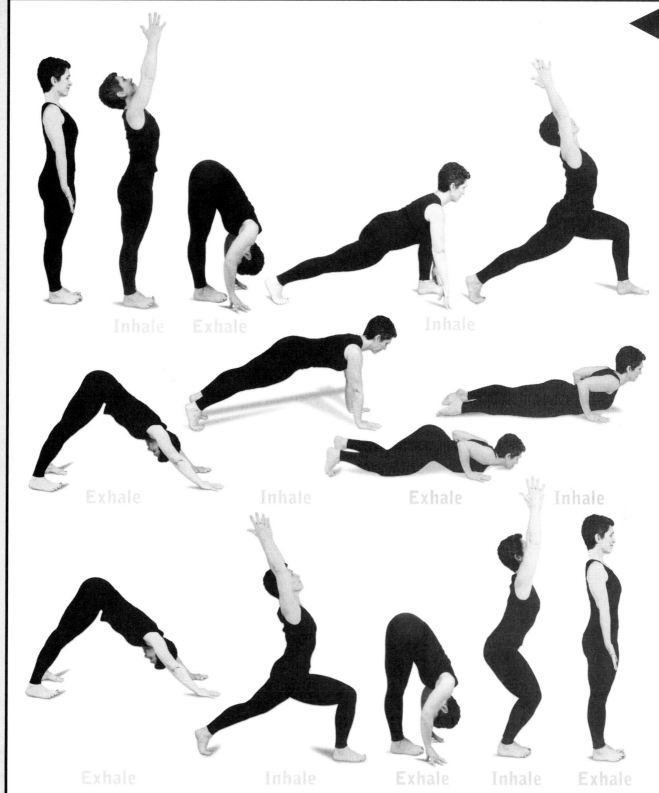

Inhale   Exhale   Inhale

Exhale   Inhale   Exhale   Inhale

Exhale   Inhale   Exhale   Inhale   Exhale

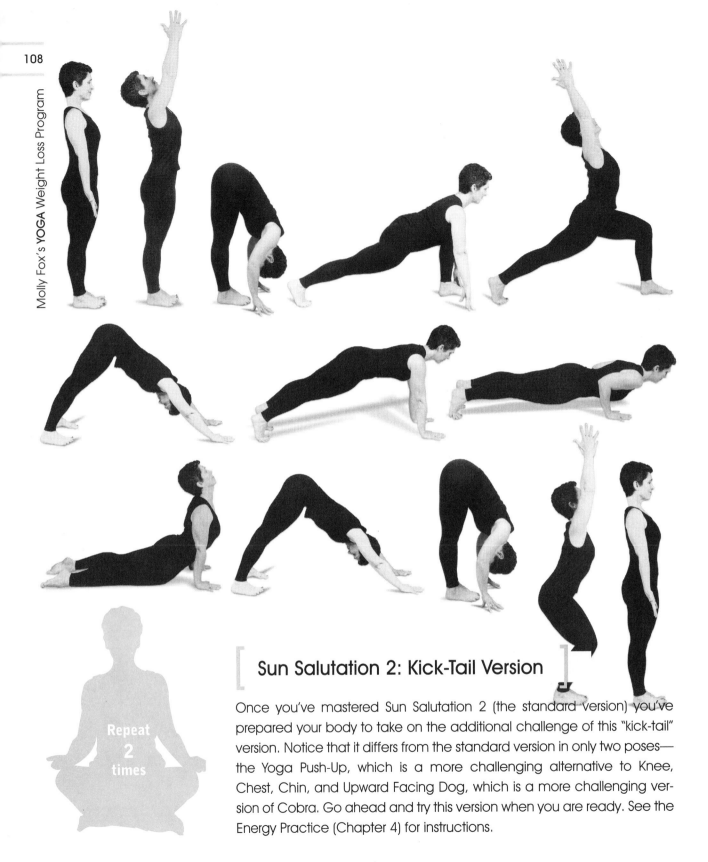

**Repeat
2
times**

Sun Salutation 2: Kick-Tail Version

Once you've mastered Sun Salutation 2 (the standard version) you've prepared your body to take on the additional challenge of this "kick-tail" version. Notice that it differs from the standard version in only two poses—the Yoga Push-Up, which is a more challenging alternative to Knee, Chest, Chin, and Upward Facing Dog, which is a more challenging version of Cobra. Go ahead and try this version when you are ready. See the Energy Practice (Chapter 4) for instructions.

Strong Leg Flow

This flow sequence focuses on strengthening the major muscle groups in the lower legs, gluteus, quadriceps, and hamstrings. Strengthening these muscles will create more muscle mass, which will burn more calories now and in the future. Burning more calories equals more weight loss! Enjoy the shake, rattle, and roll of your muscles as they develop their power. Honor your innate potential for strength and freedom.

Hold each pose for 5 full breaths. As you get stronger and you want a "kick-tail" workout, you can hold up to 1 minute, which is really intense! Continue to monitor your breathing, though. As the intensity increases, there's a tendency for the breathing to go all askew and labored, which you don't want. If this happens, just pull back on the intensity so that your breathing becomes more controlled. Think of it as a dance between intensity and breath control. As you get stronger, you will be able to control your breath better even with the greater intensity of the movement. (Remember, increasing your intensity is a very effective way to burn more calories and ultimately lose more fat.)

Give yourself a reasonable goal in the beginning. You want to make this a daily habit.

Hold each pose in the Strength Practice for 5 breaths and do 2 rounds for each of the following:

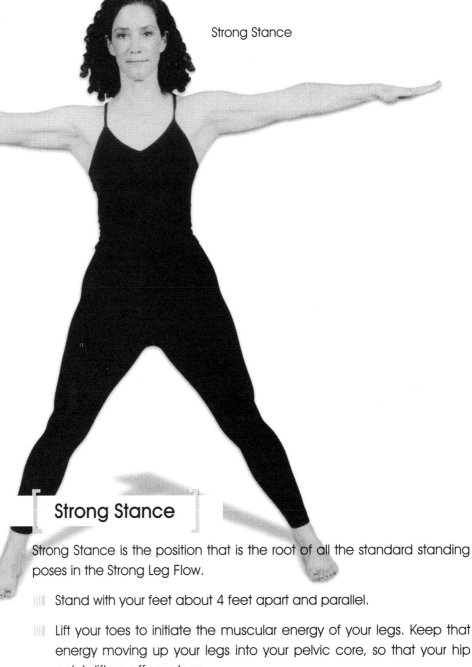

Strong Stance

5 breaths

Strong Stance

Strong Stance is the position that is the root of all the standard standing poses in the Strong Leg Flow.

|||| Stand with your feet about 4 feet apart and parallel.

|||| Lift your toes to initiate the muscular energy of your legs. Keep that energy moving up your legs into your pelvic core, so that your hip points lift up off your legs.

|||| Stretch your arms out to the sides, making muscles in your arms. As you sense the integration of your arm bones into your shoulders, broaden your collarbones and draw your shoulder blades onto your back.

|||| Extend out through all parts of your body like the radiating star that you are.

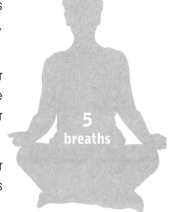

Horse

[Horse]

Horse is a dynamic pose that strengthens your legs, your buttocks, and the large muscle groups of the body. This is my favorite leg strengthening sequence: It's powerful, effective, and fun to do.

 Turn both feet out about 20 degrees. Your legs should be approximately four feet apart.

 Bend your knees and line them up over your toes, lowering your hips to a plié squat (as in ballet). Continue to press your thighbones out, maintaining the knee-over-toe relationship.

 Press firmly into the four corners of your feet, and pull up into your pelvic core. (Remember the four corners? The big toe mound, the outer ball, and both inner and outer heel.) From there, scoop your tailbone under, feeling your hip points lift.

 Press your palms together and place them at your heart in a prayer position. As your hands press together, feel how your shoulder blades feel strong on your back.

5
breaths

Wide Leg Forward Bend

This pose strengthens your legs as it stretches your back.

|||| Place your hands on the floor and bring your feet parallel, keeping your legs about 3½ to 4 feet apart as before, lining your center ankle and knee over your second toe.

|||| Press down through the four corners of your feet and lift your thigh muscles and hip points as you work toward straightening your legs. Keep your fingertips on the floor to gauge how far to straighten your legs. If you feel your back start to round, back off and bend your knees.

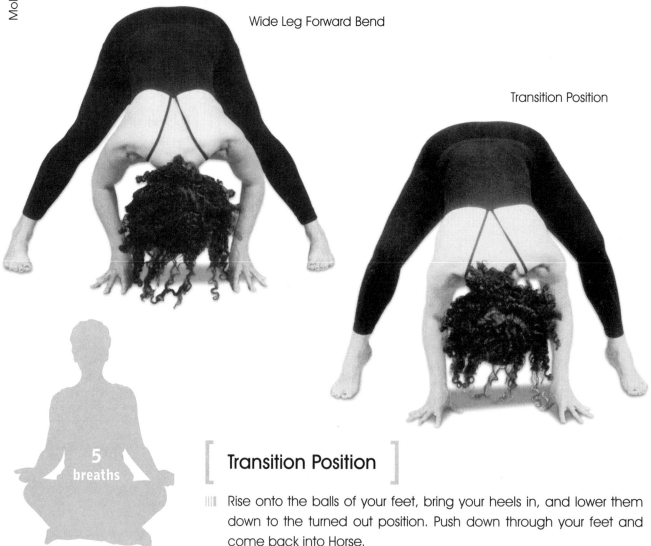

Wide Leg Forward Bend

Transition Position

5 breaths

Transition Position

|||| Rise onto the balls of your feet, bring your heels in, and lower them down to the turned out position. Push down through your feet and come back into Horse.

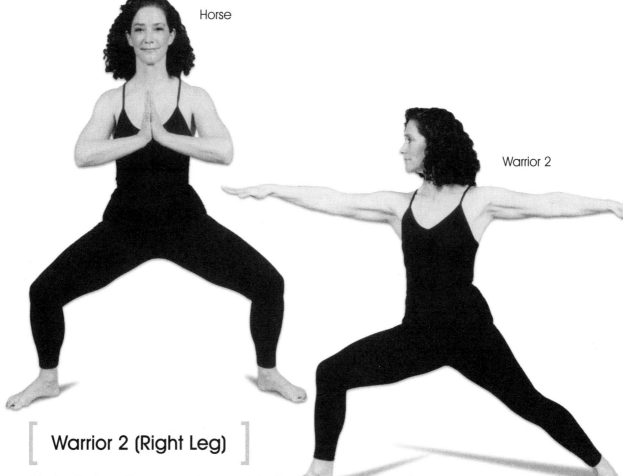

Horse

Warrior 2

[Warrior 2 (Right Leg)]

Warrior 2 strengthens your legs and buttocks and builds endurance. It's hard work, but hang in there; the payoff is huge.

- Straighten your legs from Horse. Turn your left leg in 15 degrees and your right leg out 90 degrees.

- From the four corners of your feet, pull your leg muscles up and into your pelvic core. Move your inner groin back, and then scoop your tailbone under. You will feel a lift in your hip points.

- Keeping this lift in your hip points, move your right shinbone forward so that your knee is at a 90-degree angle over the center of your foot and in line with your toes.

- Make your arm muscles strong, so that you feel your arm bones integrate into your shoulder socket. This will broaden your collarbones and lay your shoulder blades flat on your back.

- Feel the strength, power, and freedom of the Warrior.

5
breaths

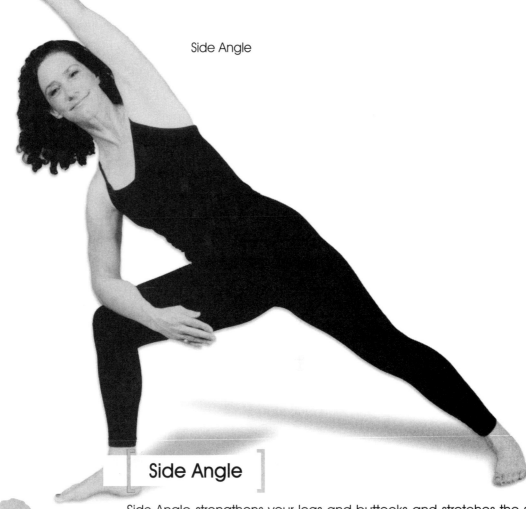

Side Angle

Side Angle

5 breaths

Side Angle strengthens your legs and buttocks and stretches the side of your torso.

▥ Keeping the strength of Warrior 2, extend both sides of your waist out to the right and lay your right forearm on your right thighbone.

▥ Bring your left arm forward in front of your shoulder. Make muscles in your arms and move your arm bone into your back so you can feel your shoulder blade lie flat on your back. Keeping that feeling of your shoulder blade lying flat on your back, sweep your arm over your head.

▥ Experience the uplifting stretch sensation in your chest.

High Lunge

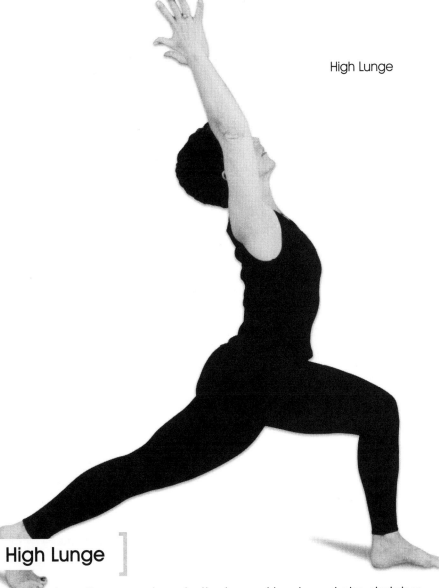

High Lunge

This Lunge strengthens your legs, buttocks, and back, and also stretches the side of your body.

||| From Side Angle, bring both hands onto your front thigh. Pivot onto the ball of your back foot and bring it parallel with your front foot.

||| From the strength of your feet, draw energy up to your pelvic core and lift your hip points up off your pelvis.

||| Sweep your arms out and up alongside your ears.

||| Experience the stability of your arms into your back as your chest expands up to the sky from strong legs.

5
breaths

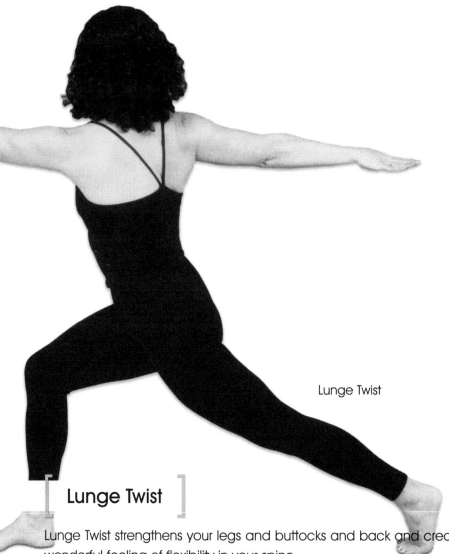

Lunge Twist

[Lunge Twist]

Lunge Twist strengthens your legs and buttocks and back and creates a wonderful feeling of flexibility in your spine.

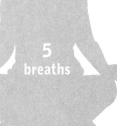

5 breaths

||||| Keeping the leg and core strength of the Lunge, bring your arms out to the side.

||||| Firm your hips into the bones and revolve your rib cage around into the twist.

||||| Firm your arms as you expand your collarbones and reach out through your fingertips. Turn your head and look at the hand behind you, keeping your neck free and your throat soft.

||||| Feel your twist come from strong and stable legs. Twist up from your legs, up and out through your head as if you were the moving colors on a barbershop pole.

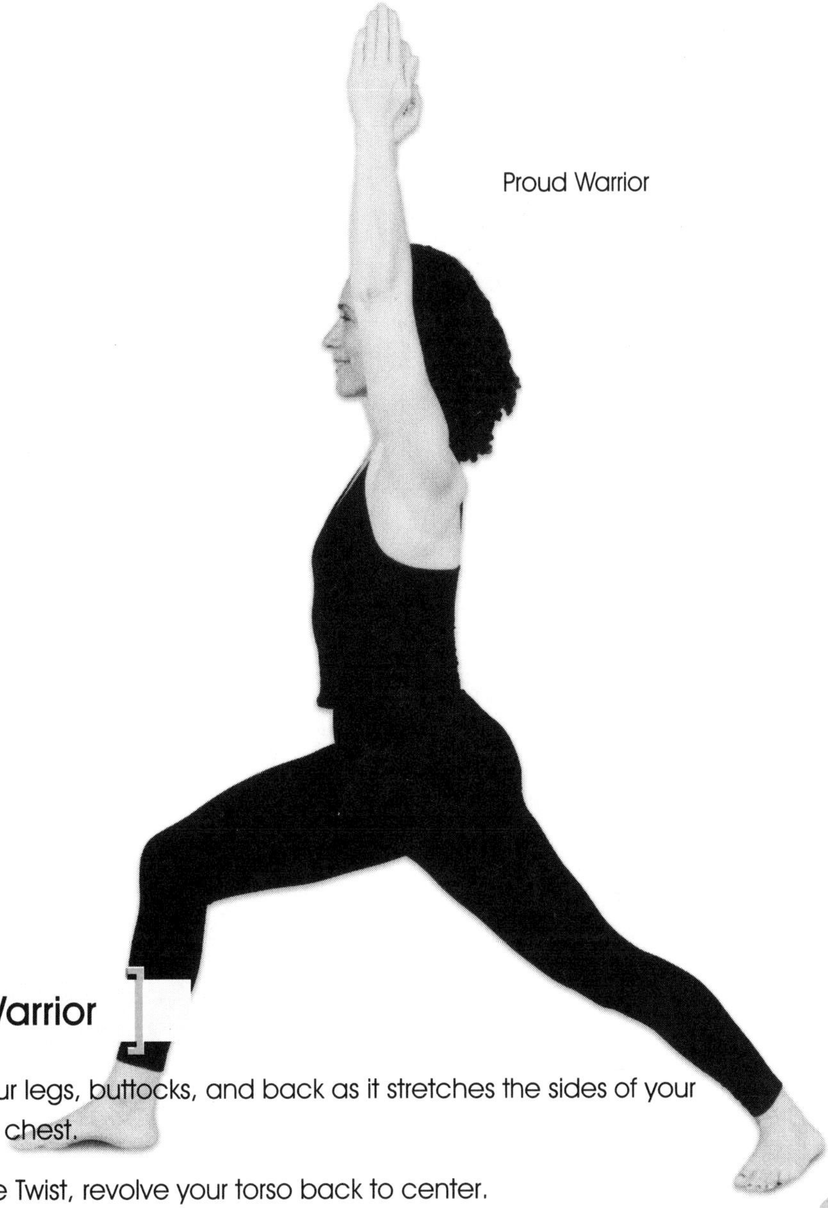

Proud Warrior

[Proud Warrior]

Strengthens your legs, buttocks, and back as it stretches the sides of your body and your chest.

▎ From Lunge Twist, revolve your torso back to center.

▎ Sweep your arms out and up alongside your ears, and straighten your right leg. Revolve your left foot out 15 degrees, and lower your left heel.

▎ From the four corners of your feet, draw your muscles into your legs and up to your pelvic core.

▎ Keeping the lift of your hip points, move your right shinbone forward until your knee is bent to a 90-degree angle, with your knee over the center of your foot and lined up with your toes.

▎ As you stand strong, feel the pride that comes with strengthening your body.

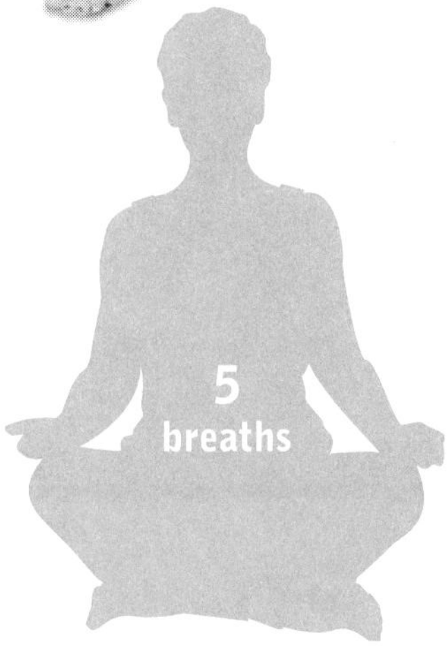

5 breaths

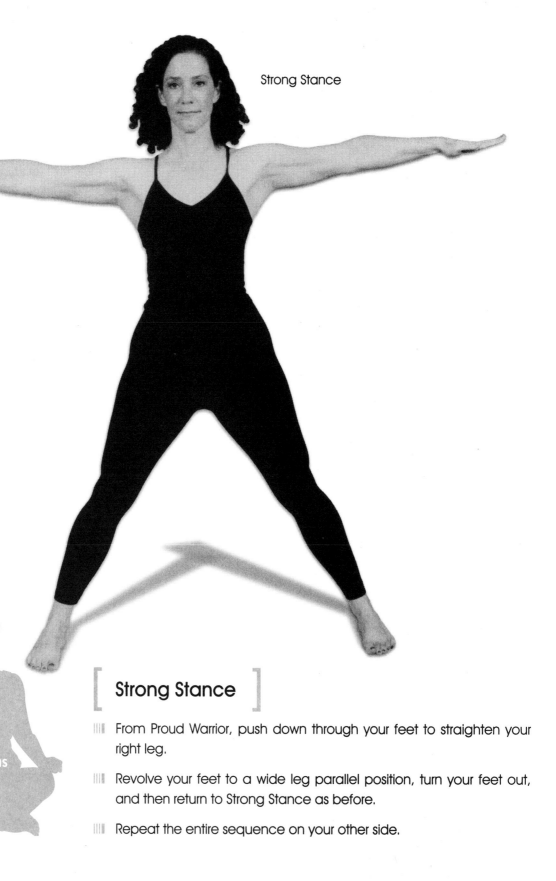

Strong Stance

5 breaths

[Strong Stance]

|||| From Proud Warrior, push down through your feet to straighten your right leg.

|||| Revolve your feet to a wide leg parallel position, turn your feet out, and then return to Strong Stance as before.

|||| Repeat the entire sequence on your other side.

Strong Back Flow

In this sequence we return to the rhythmic and holding sequences that were introduced in Chapter 4. Strong Back Flow will strengthen your back muscles and give you the physical power to sit and stand up straight. We spend a lot of time bending forward, working on our computers and even picking up the kids; we also need to spend some time bending backward. Psychologically you can think of it as gaining a strong backbone. (Now there's something that everyone could use!)

Back problems plague a large percentage of the population and prevent free and easy movement, limiting the ability to do exercise effectively. By strengthening the back you reduce the chances of injury and pain and increase your ability to exercise at full capacity, leading to far more calorie burning and far more fat loss.

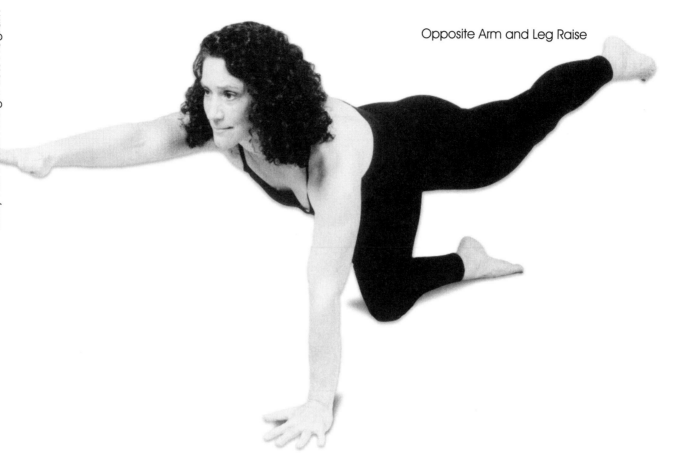

Opposite Arm and Leg Raise

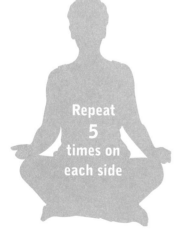

**Repeat
5
times on
each side**

[Opposite Arm and Leg Raise]

This sequence strengthens your back and buttocks, increases your coordination and balance, and tones your abdominals.

|||| Get on all fours. Firm the muscles of your arms, legs, and belly.

|||| Keeping your pelvic core strength, inhale as you raise your left arm and your right leg.

|||| As you raise your left arm and right leg, keep your chest stretching forward and your hip points lifting up.

|||| Exhale as you lower down and do the other side.

|||| Repeat 5 times on each side.

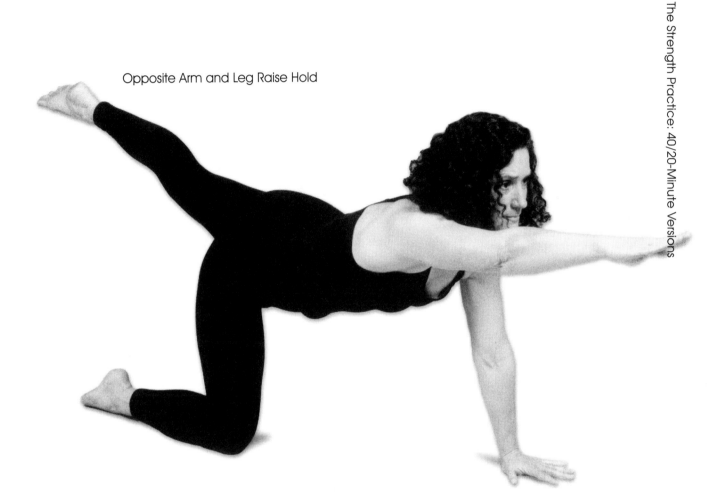

Opposite Arm and Leg Raise Hold

[**Opposite Arm and Leg Raise Hold**]

Holding this pose creates dynamic strength.

|||| Hold your right arm and left leg up for up to 5 breaths.

|||| Exhale, lower down, and repeat on the other side.

|||| Kick-tail version—hold up to 1 minute. Keep your pelvic core lifted.

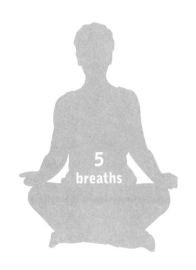

5 breaths

Locust

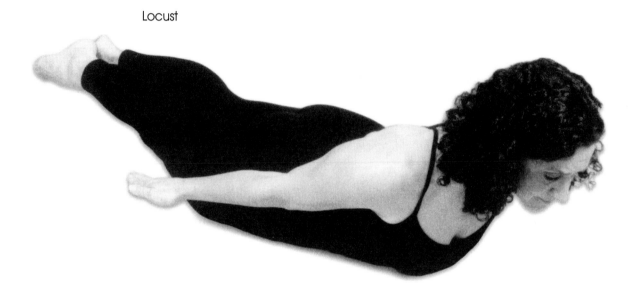

[Locust]

Locust Pose strengthens your back, buttocks, and legs—the whole back side of your body.

▸ Lie on your belly.

▸ Bring your inner ankles together and your arms down by your sides with your palms up.

▸ Firm your muscles into the bones and draw energy up to your pelvic core, lifting your hip points up toward your chest.

▸ Inhale as you lift your legs, chest, arms, and head off the floor, stretching your chest and legs away from your center. Keep your neck long.

▸ Exhale as you lower down.

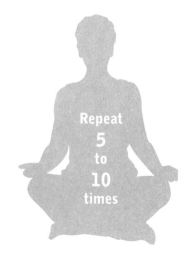

Repeat
5
to
10
times

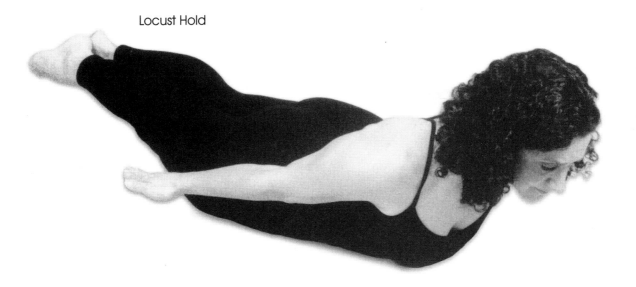

Locust Hold

[Locust Hold]

Holding this pose will intensify the strengthening effects of the Locust Pose.

▥ On your last lift hold for up to 5 full, deep breaths.

▥ Exhale; lower down.

▥ Kick-tail version: hold up to 1 minute, but maintain hip point lift and abdominal strength.

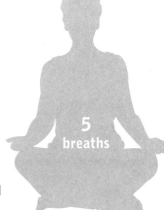

5
breaths

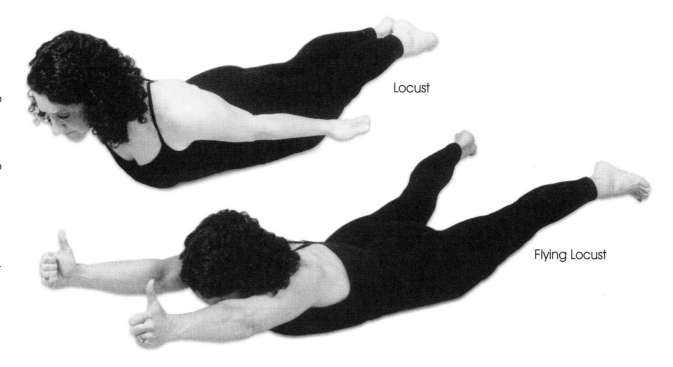

Locust

Flying Locust

[Flying Locust]

This rhythmic pose will strengthen your outer hips, buttocks, and particularly your upper back.

||| Return to Locust Hold.

||| While keeping the muscles of your entire body pulled up and into your pelvic core, keep your chest lifted and your collarbones broad (Locust).

||| Inhale as you open your legs apart; sweep your arms around and forward up near your ears with your thumbs up like you are hitchhiking (Flying Locust).

||| With your arms in this position, relax your upper back muscles, and hold your arms up with your lower shoulder blade muscles. This may take a while to get, but keep at it. It will strengthen these notoriously weak muscles, which are responsible for drawing your shoulder blades down your back. Strengthening these muscles will make sitting more pleasurable.

||| Exhale as you bring your arms back by your side and draw your legs together. Keep your legs high as you move them.

||| Sit back into Child's Pose (page 51).

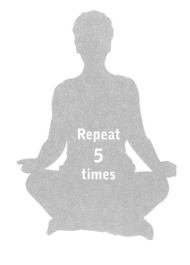

Repeat
5
times

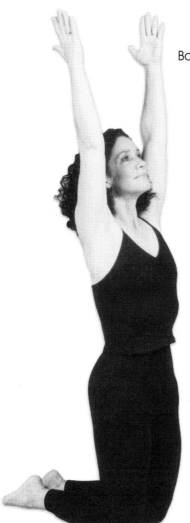

Back Release Inhale

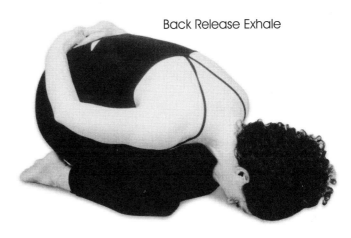

Back Release Exhale

[Back Release]

After the Strong Back Flow sequence you will want to stretch out your back. This is a terrific way to do it. You will strengthen your abdominal muscles at the same time as you stretch out the lower back, and it will feel great.

▥ From Child's Pose (page 51), inhale as you come onto your knees, sweeping your arms up by your ears (Back Release Inhale).

▥ Exhale as you draw your pelvic core up and in and sit back onto your heels. Your arms will sweep back onto your lower back as you fold over and bring your head to the floor (Back Release Exhale).

▥ Maintain a steady lift in your belly as your sit on your heels.

Repeat
10
times

Strong Core Flow

This dynamic flow sequence will strengthen your abdominals for core support. This means it will assist in keeping your posture tall and your back stable. When you exhale during this sequence, draw your pelvic core (deep belly muscles) up and in. This action will help you keep your balance. This continues to be a favorite series in my classes.

Forearm Plank

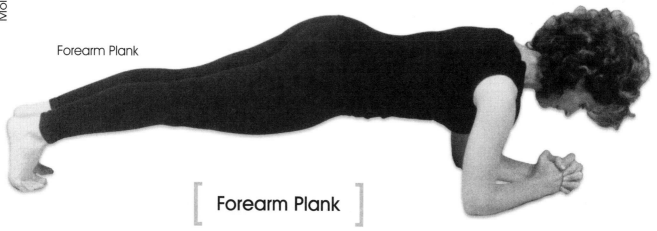

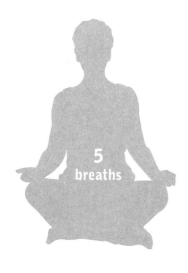

5 breaths

[Forearm Plank]

This strengthens your whole body, particularly your abdominals. It also develops core stability.

Developing core stability makes your waist appear smaller and gives you a longer, leaner look. Think of how ballet dancers stand and walk erect, long, lean, and pulled up with tight abdominals. This is core stability at its best-looking.

|||| From all fours (on your hands and knees), come onto your forearms and lace your fingers together as if you are holding hands with yourself.

|||| Curl your toes under and straighten your knees so that your body comes into a plank position.

|||| Tighten or firm all your muscles and pull that strength into your pelvic core. Then press down and out through your feet and forearms to become lighter.

|||| Hold for 5 breaths.

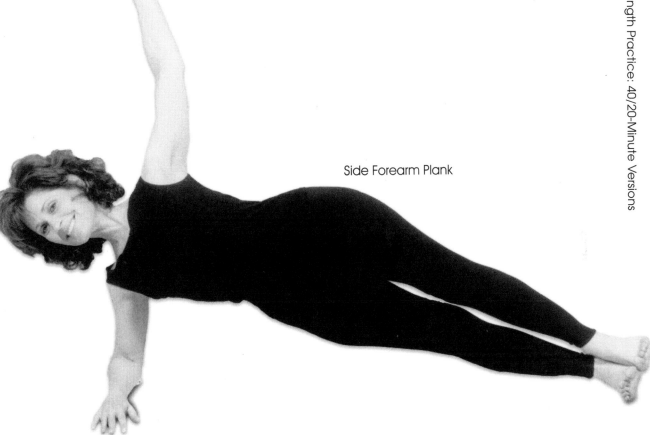

Side Forearm Plank

[Side Forearm Plank]

Side Forearm Planks strengthen your oblique muscles (the abdominal muscles at the sides of the body, right under the "love handles"). It increases balance and core stability.

▥ From Forearm Plank, roll over to your right forearm and onto the outside of your right foot. Place your left foot on top of your right, and flex both feet.

▥ Lift your hips up so that you feel a contraction in the muscles on the side of your waist (your oblique muscles).

▥ Hold for 5 breaths.

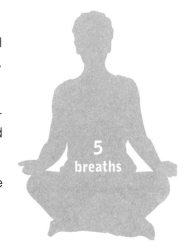

5 breaths

[Forearm Plank]

||| Return to Forearm Plank.

||| Hold for 5 breaths.

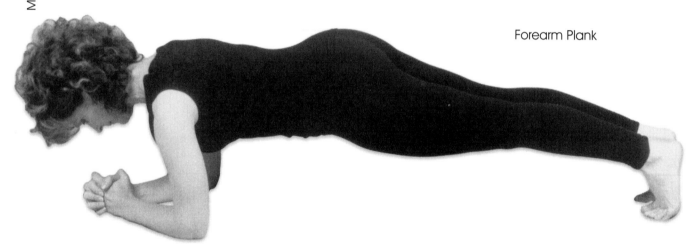

Forearm Plank

5 breaths each

[Side Forearm Plank]

||| Repeat Side Forearm Plank (page 127) on your left side.

||| Hold for 5 breaths.

||| Return through Forearm Plank and release into Child's Pose (page 51).

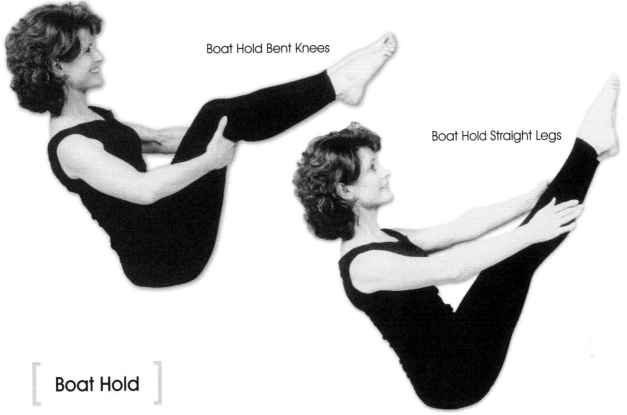

Boat Hold Bent Knees

Boat Hold Straight Legs

[Boat Hold]

A Boat Hold strengthens your back, your abdominals, and your legs.

By toning and tightening the abdominals you can gradually teach yourself to walk with these muscles pulled in and up, which can immediately reduce the size of your waistline.

- From a seated position, lean back onto your fingertips.
- Bend your knees. Draw your legs into your chest keeping your toes on the floor.
- Keep your chest lifted and continue to funnel energy into your pelvic core. Keeping your chest lifted, bring your toes off the floor and straighten your legs up toward the ceiling. Extend your arms out in front of you (Boat Hold Straight Knees). If this is too challenging, bend your knees at a 90-degree angle (Boat Hold Bent Knees), or return your toes to the floor.
- Lift your heart courageously as you charter new territory.
- For a kick-tail choice, repeat up to 5 times.

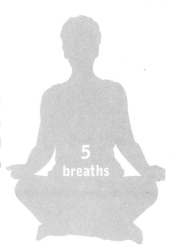

5
breaths

Twist for Strength (right side)

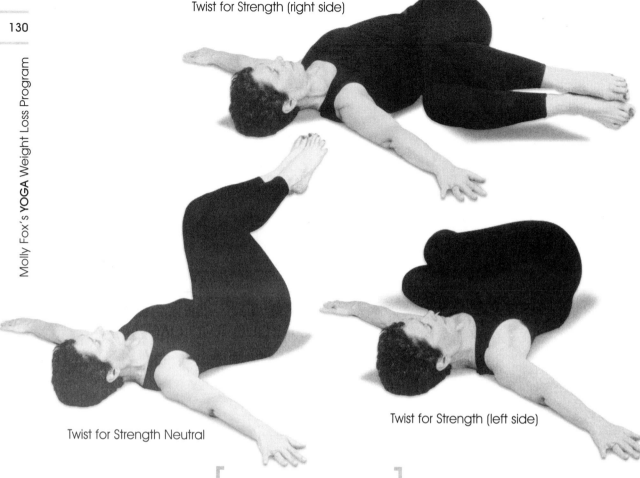

Twist for Strength Neutral

Twist for Strength (left side)

[Twist for Strength]

The twist strengthens your abdominal muscles.

||||| Lie on your back.

||||| Drawing your knees into your chest, lay your arms out to the sides on the floor (Twist for Strength Neutral).

||||| Keep your chest lifted and throat soft.

||||| Inhale as you take your legs to the right side until they are 1 inch off the floor (right side photo).

||||| Exhale as you draw your navel in, bringing your legs back to center.

||||| Inhale as you take your legs to the left side until they are 1 inch off the floor (left side photo).

||||| Exhale as you draw your navel in, bringing your legs back to center.

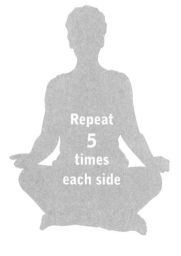

**Repeat
5
times
each side**

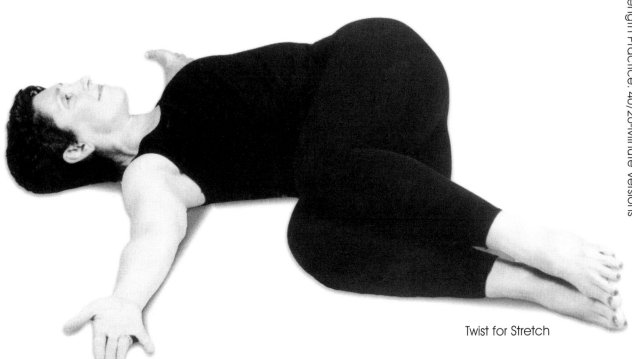

Twist for Stretch

[Twist for Stretch]

This twist stretches your back, hips, and chest.

▌▌▌ On your last repetition of Twist for Strength to either side, bring your legs to the ground.

▌▌▌ Hold for a minimum of 5 breaths. Let your body release.

▌▌▌ Repeat on the other side.

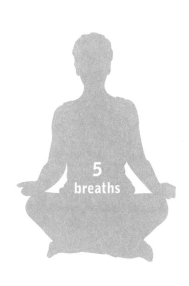

5
breaths

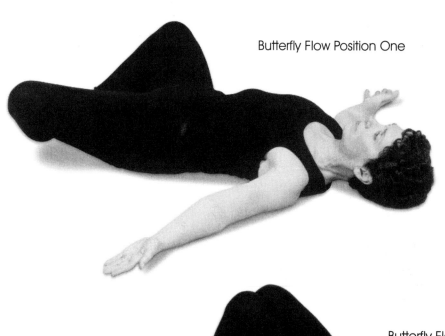

Butterfly Flow Position One

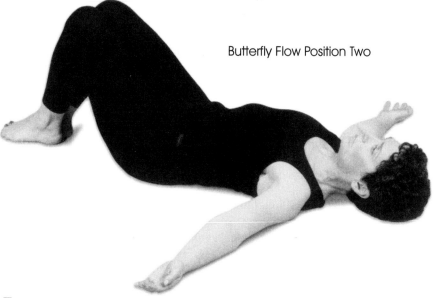

Butterfly Flow Position Two

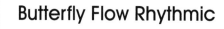

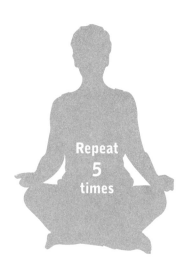

**Repeat
5
times**

[Butterfly Flow Rhythmic]

This releases tightness in your hips and creates a sense of ease in your movement.

|||| Lie on your back with the soles of your feet together, knees open, and feet about 12 inches away from your pelvis (Position One).

|||| Take about 3 breaths to slowly bring your knees together and your feet flat on the floor (about 10 seconds each repetition) (Position Two).

|||| Return to original position.

[Butterfly Flow Hold]

Holding Butterfly Flow stretches your groin by allowing gravity to do its work and assist in stretching your inner thighs.

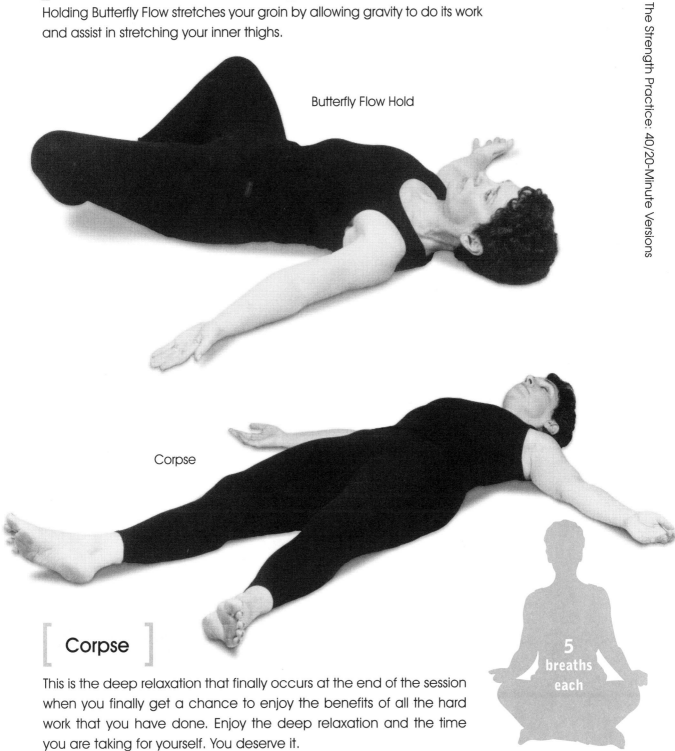

Butterfly Flow Hold

Corpse

5
breaths
each

[Corpse]

This is the deep relaxation that finally occurs at the end of the session when you finally get a chance to enjoy the benefits of all the hard work that you have done. Enjoy the deep relaxation and the time you are taking for yourself. You deserve it.

On Your Back Breathing

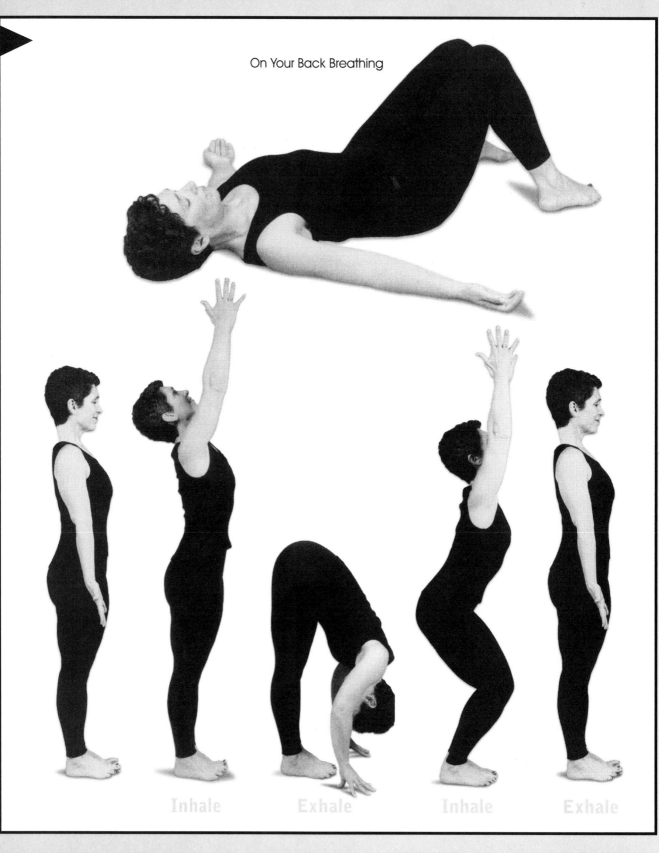

Inhale   Exhale   Inhale   Exhale

After Sun Salutation 1, do two rounds of either Sun Salutation 2: Standard Version or Sun Salutation 2: Kick-Tail Version.

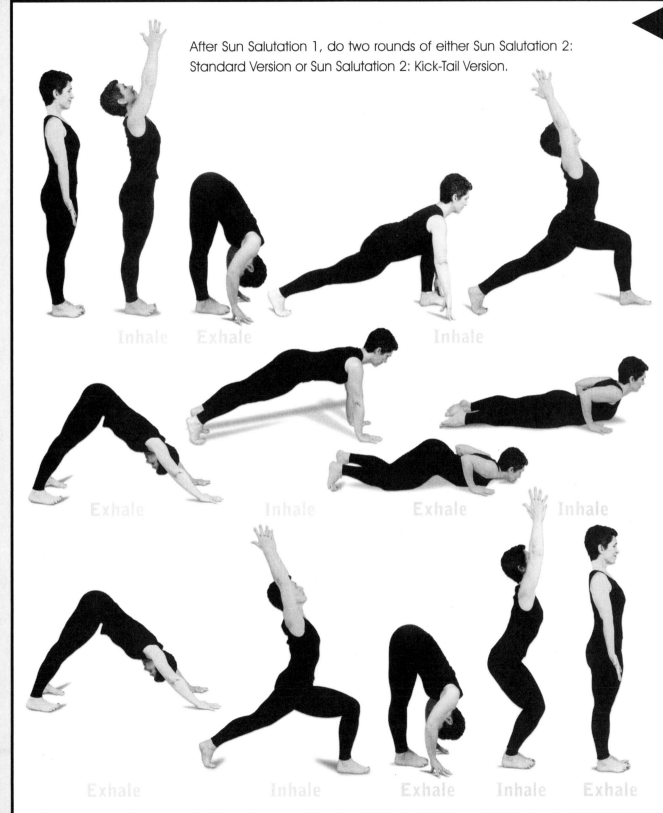

Inhale   Exhale   Inhale

Exhale   Inhale   Exhale   Inhale

Exhale   Inhale   Exhale   Inhale   Exhale

Repeat 2 times

Repeat sequence on other side for one round.

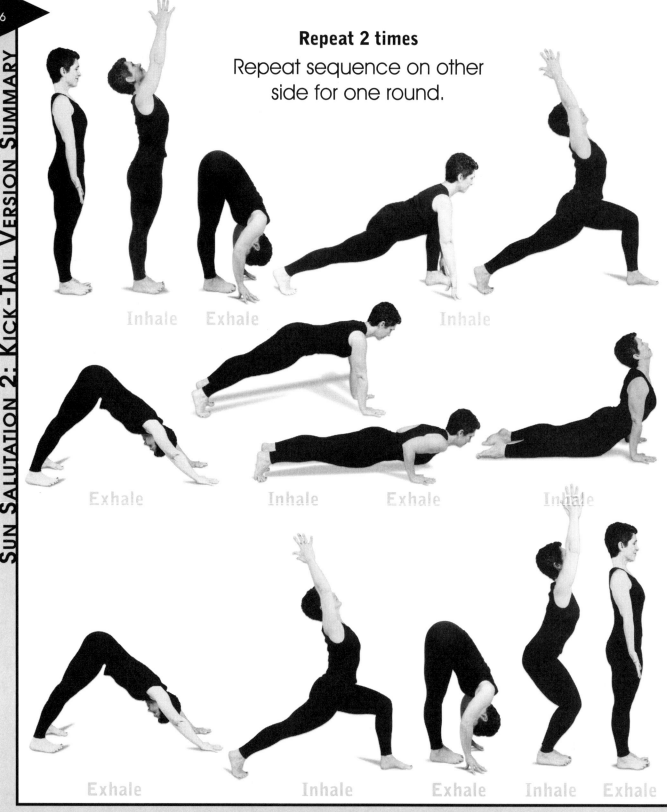

Inhale   Exhale   Inhale

Exhale   Inhale   Exhale   Inhale

Exhale   Inhale   Exhale   Inhale   Exhale

Repeat 2 times

Repeat sequence on other side, then repeat whole sequence again.

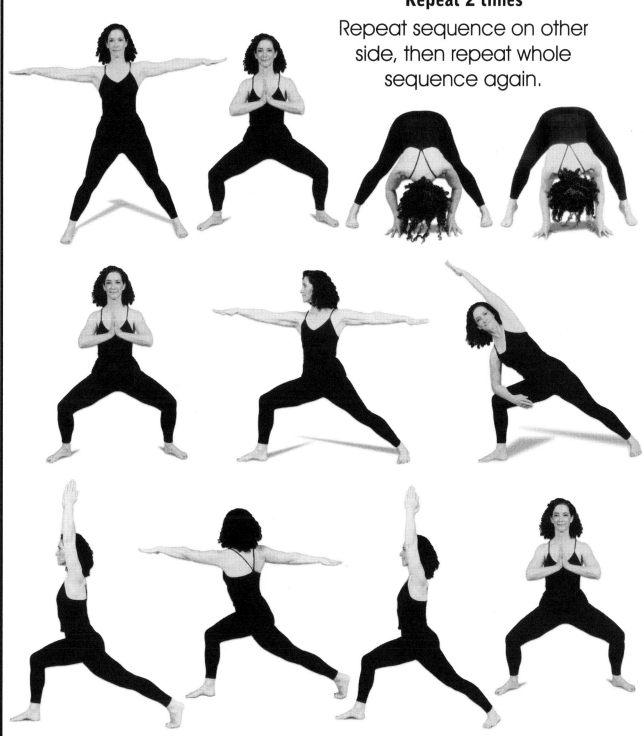

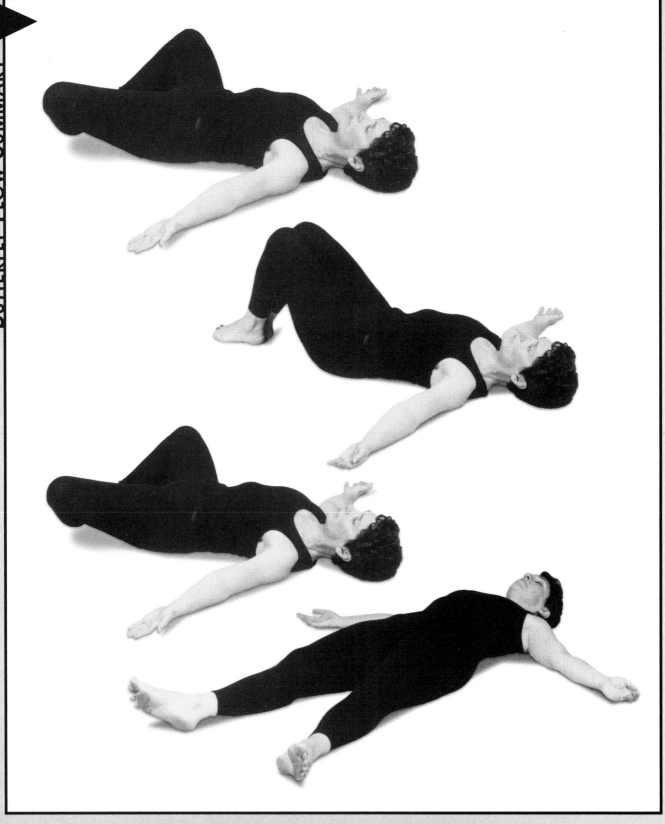

Strength Practice Summary

The Strength Practices in this chapter will have a profound effect on all the muscles of your body: your legs, back, chest, arms, and core abdominal muscles. Their purpose is to increase muscular development, which will in turn decrease body fat. By doing it on a regular basis you will increase your metabolic rate and become a more efficient "fat-burning machine." When we're stronger, we move through all of our daily activities more easily and efficiently, which leads naturally to us being more active.

When it's easier to move, you move more. It's as simple as that. Move more in your daily life and you will see weight dropping off naturally.

Now let's move on to some stress-reducing sequences that will help you relax and improve your mood: the Calming Practice.

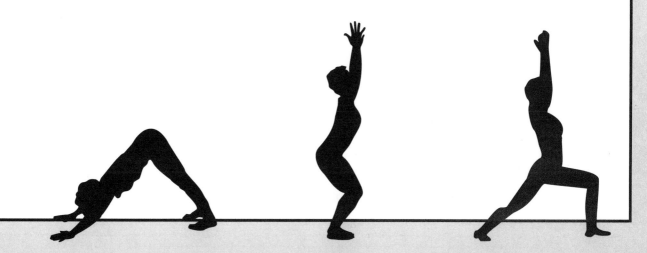

Chapter Six
The Calming Practice:
40/20-Minute Versions

How did the rose ever open
its heart and give to this
world all its beauty? It felt
the encouragement of light
against its being. Otherwise,
we all remain too frightened.

—Hafiz, Sufi poet

The Calming Practice, known as Yin Yoga, is designed to relax you while at the same time releasing chronic holding patterns in the connective tissue of your body. According to ancient Chinese Meridian Theory, chi (or life force) runs through all of the connective tissue in our bodies. It can be restricted by habitual holding patterns that are created just in the process of living life.

A Yang Yoga Practice, which is like the Energy and Strength practices, primarily affects the muscles and makes them stronger and more efficient. The activity is based on rhythmic motion and shorter holdings.

In the Yin practice, you will notice the holding time for each pose is longer. We do this so that the deeper, denser connective can be affected and renewed.

According to Paul Grilley in his book *Yin Yoga: Outline of a Quiet Practice,* the fundamental characteristic of Yin Yoga is holding poses for several minutes. Connective tissue doesn't respond to brief rhythmical stretches the way muscles do. Connective tissues are tough and fibrous and stretch best when pulled like taffy. Holding postures for a few minutes with moderate stress is not going to stretch the connective tissue to the breaking point; it is only going to stretch it minutely.

If you are persistent, the body will respond by making the tissue a little longer and thicker—which is exactly what you want.

The Calming Practice—in addition to being a marvelous tool for rejuvenation and self-awareness—has a practical effect on weight loss in two ways. The first is that it lowers stress hormones, which, as you learned in Chapter 2, are a major player in weight gain, particularly around the abdominal area. Second, becoming calm and freeing up your body to move more efficiently and with more freedom will give you the green light to be more active all day. Voilà!! More activity = weight loss. I have found that giving myself permission to relax completely gives birth to a natural desire to move. After all, it is our nature.

Yin vs. Yang

The Calming Practice (Yin style) is very different from the Energy and Strength practices (Yang style) in Chapters 4 and 5. In the Yin style your muscles will feel completely relaxed, which is very different from the feeling you get when you are practicing for energy and strength. It's important to know the key elements of practicing in this more relaxed way.

- Relax your muscles in each pose so that the deeper connective tissue will be affected. (It is not possible for all the muscles to completely relax, but work conscientiously to relax as best you can.)
- The forward bending poses in this series can be held for longer periods, as you will see by the times given in the practice.
- Breathe naturally and find a soft edge. A soft edge is where you can comfortably hold the pose and still feel a stretch for the stated period of time.
- If you cannot hold the pose, it is fine to come out of the pose, take some time, and then return. This can be done as often as necessary. Your ability to stay in the pose will improve with practice.
- You can prop yourself up in some of the poses using a block, pillow, or bolster. I have used them all, but my favorite is the cushion from the back of the couch! It's just the right density. So don't be afraid to improvise.

The 40-Minute Yin Practice

This longer practice is so delicious and deeply relaxing that the time will fly by. When it's over you'll feel rejuvenated, refreshed, and calm.

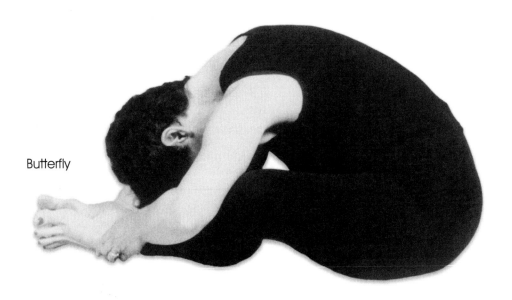

Butterfly

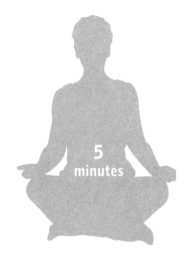

5 minutes

[Butterfly]

This pose is a soft, quiet one that stretches the lower spine and groin. Feel free to let your thoughts move inward, and focus on your breath.

- Sit with your feet about 12 to 16 inches away from your pelvis, and fold over.

- If you like, or if you feel any strain or discomfort, fill in the space between your feet, the floor, and your head with a pillow or bolster. This will allow you to relax deeper into the pose.

Seal: Level One

Seal: Level Two

[Seal]

Seal Pose is the queen pose of your lower back and sacral area. The practice of this pose will increase your lumbar curve and strengthen your lower back, as well as help you sit taller and walk with more grace.

The Seal Pose took me a while to get used to, but now it is my favorite. It feels like a self-massage. Remember that it's important to stay at your "soft edge" so your muscles can stay relaxed. Go easy on yourself. Whenever you feel uncomfortable or stressed, back off and do the Level One position.

- Lie on your belly and bring your elbows underneath your shoulders. Let your legs be parallel and relaxed. Let your spine move into your body, particularly your lower back and upper buttocks (Level One).

- When you're comfortable with the beginning position, straighten your arms and hold for the duration (Level Two).

3 to 5 minutes

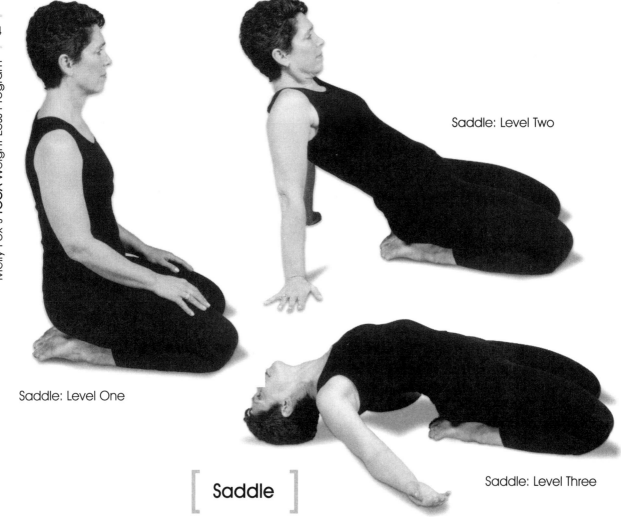

Saddle: Level Two

Saddle: Level One

Saddle: Level Three

[Saddle]

The Saddle Pose is another wonderful pose to strengthen your sacral and lumbar area, assisting you in standing and sitting taller. You will also stretch and release tension in your groin and the front of your pelvis. Start easy and build up to Level Three. It may take a while, but the payoff—freedom of movement—will be well worth it.

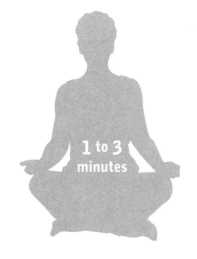

1 to 3 minutes

|||| Sit on your heels with your knees 6 to 12 inches apart. If this is all you can do for now, hold this (Level One). If you want to take it to the next level, walk back onto your hands (Level Two). For even more stretch, lower down onto your elbows. In the final pose, the top of your head will be on the floor (Level Three).

|||| Remember the soft edge. That edge will shift quickly in Saddle, so don't rush it.

|||| To come up, push down with your legs and hands and lift your chest.

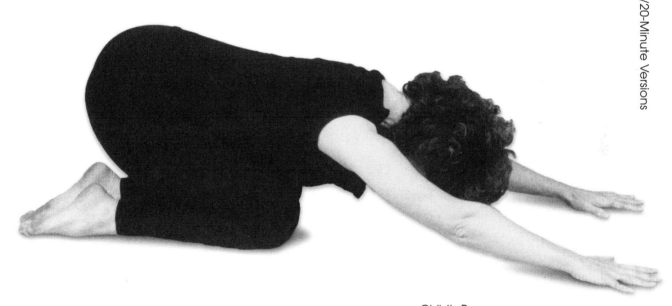

Child's Pose

[Child's Pose]

The Child's Pose will release and stretch your lower back. It is a welcome counter-pose to Seal and Saddle and a nice gentle release after backbends.

▥ Sit on your heels with your knees 6 inches apart, and bend forward.

▥ The Half Butterfly Pose stretches the back of your straight leg and the opposite section of the lower back. I love this pose

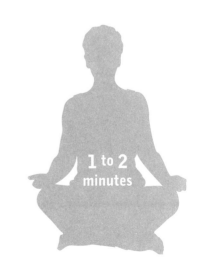

1 to 2 minutes

Half Butterfly

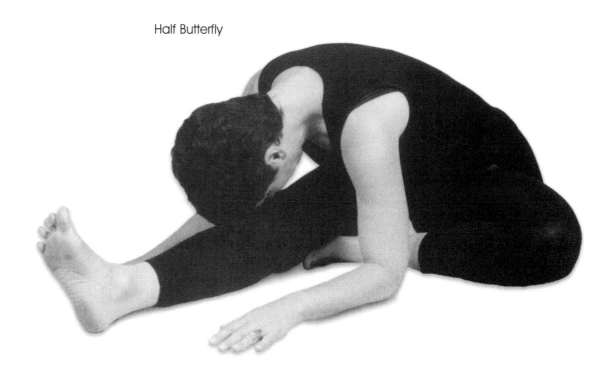

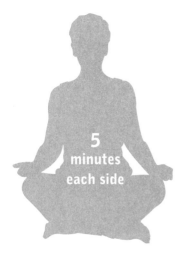

**5
minutes
each side**

[Half Butterfly]

and use it as a mini-meditation. Feel free to bolster up your body to make it even more enjoyable.

||| Extend one leg forward and bring the other foot into your inner thigh.

||| Reach forward toward the foot of your straight leg, and stretch. Your "straight" leg may very well be bent—that is perfectly okay. Feel free to use your arms for light support to hold you in the pose.

||| Release and do the same on the other leg.

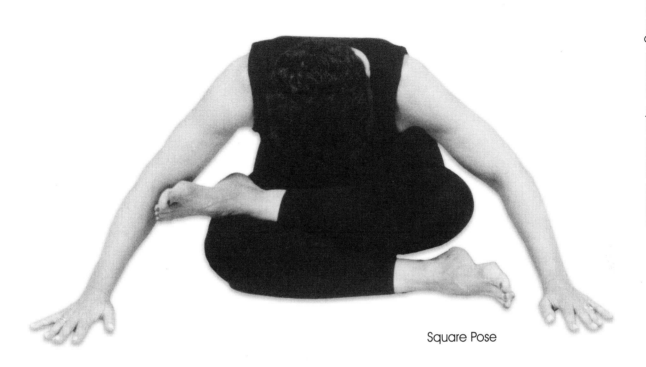

Square Pose

[Square Pose]

The Square Pose is the one I love to hate! It is intense at first, but, done consistently, becomes easier. Ultimately you will feel that the experience of doing it is totally awesome. You'll experience more freedom in your back and hips, and all of your yoga poses will become easier. The Square Pose releases and stretches lower back and hips.

|||| Sit with your legs at a square with your hips. Your left ankle will be over your right knee, and your right knee will be over your left ankle. The top knee may be higher than shown and with practice you will see it lower.

|||| Come forward as comfort allows.

|||| Feel free to come in and out of this pose, as you need.

|||| Release and repeat, reversing the top and bottom legs.

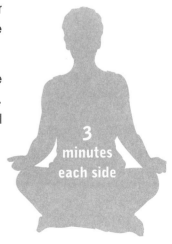

3
minutes
each side

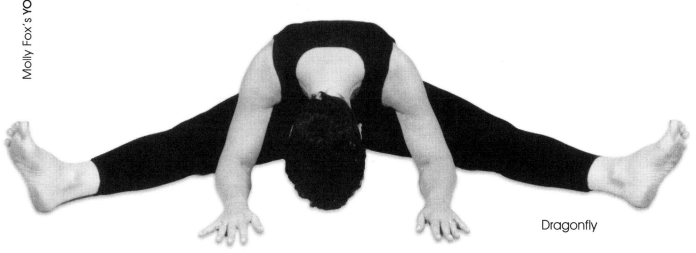

Dragonfly

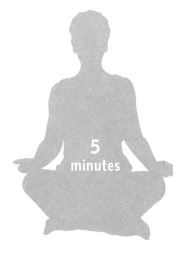

5 minutes

[Dragonfly]

Let yourself go when doing the Dragonfly. I have actually fallen asleep in this pose (much to the chagrin of my class!). You may enjoy propping yourself up in this pose with a pillow or a cushion. The Dragonfly stretches your hamstrings, groin, and lower back.

|||| Sit with your legs wide. Relax your legs, and fold over placing your hands on the floor in front of you. Your hands can offer a light support.

|||| Feel free to fill in the space between your head and the floor with a blanket, pillow, or block.

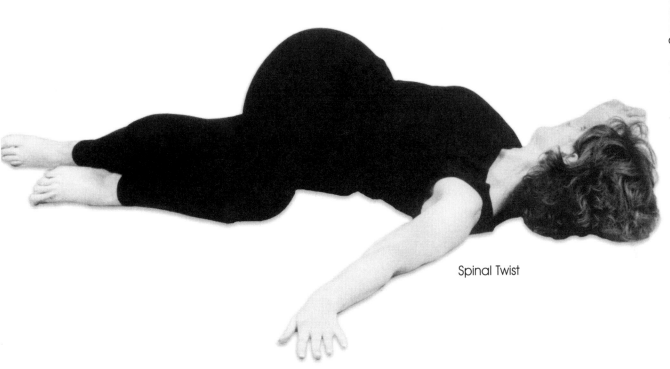

Spinal Twist

[Spinal Twist]

Yummy, yummy, yummy! After all the previous releasing and letting go, the Spinal Twist is the tiramisu of poses. Aaaahhhh . . . The Spinal Twist stretches and releases the area around your spine. If it is uncomfortable for you to cross your legs in this pose, don't cross them. Instead, just bring them both over to the side, one on top of the other.

▥ Lie on your back and bring your knees into your chest. Cross your right leg over your left (not just the ankles, your whole leg!), and then take your legs to the floor on your left side. Make sure your knees line up with your belly.

▥ Stretch your arms to the side, open your chest, and look away from your legs.

▥ Release and repeat to the other side.

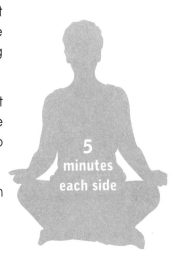

5
minutes
each side

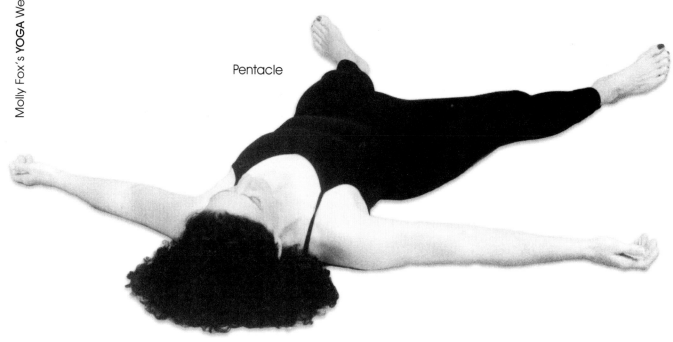

Pentacle

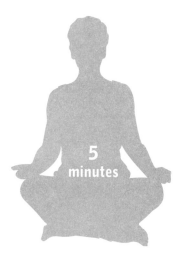

5 minutes

[**Pentacle**]

This pose is like the Corpse Pose. Completely let go and release into the floor. Give yourself the pleasure of being stress-free. Let the beautiful you shine!

|||| Lie on your back with your legs and arms open wide.

|||| Release completely into the floor, relax, and be at peace.

|||| Relax your jaw and throat, and breathe freely.

20-Minute Version

This is a wonderful midday, before-bed or "whenever-you-find-the-time-or-have-the-need" practice. Think of it as a quick "calm-down."

Butterfly

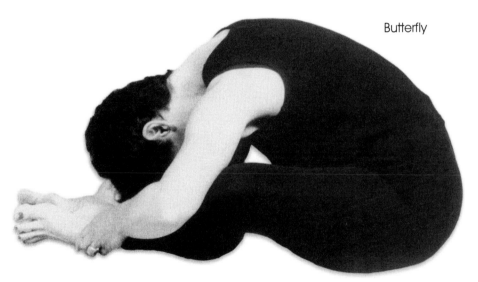

[Butterfly]

Butterfly stretches the lower spine and groin.

▥ Sit with your feet about 12 to 16 inches away from your pelvis, and fold over.

▥ If you like, fill in the space between your feet, the floor, and your head with a pillow.

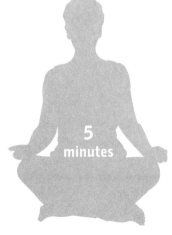

5
minutes

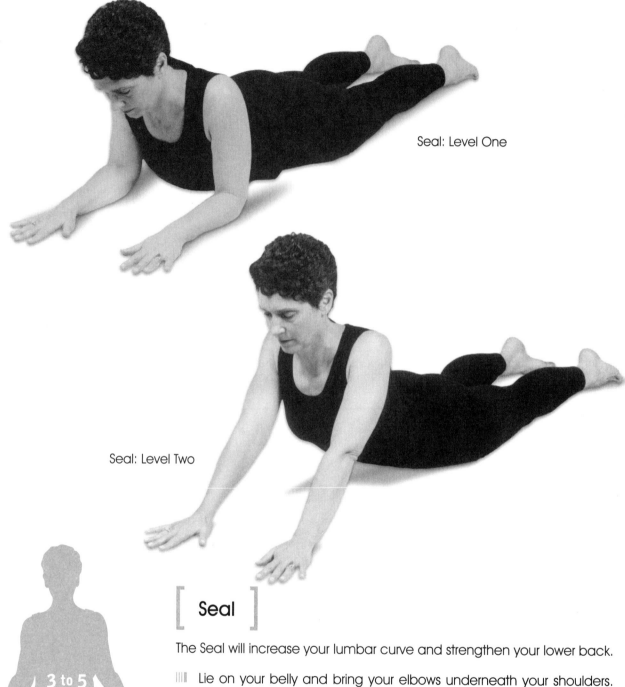

Seal: Level One

Seal: Level Two

3 to 5 minutes

[Seal]

The Seal will increase your lumbar curve and strengthen your lower back.

▥ Lie on your belly and bring your elbows underneath your shoulders. Let your legs be parallel and relaxed. Let your spine move into your body, particularly your lower back and upper buttocks (Level One).

▥ When you're comfortable with the beginning position, straighten your arms and hold for the duration (Level Two).

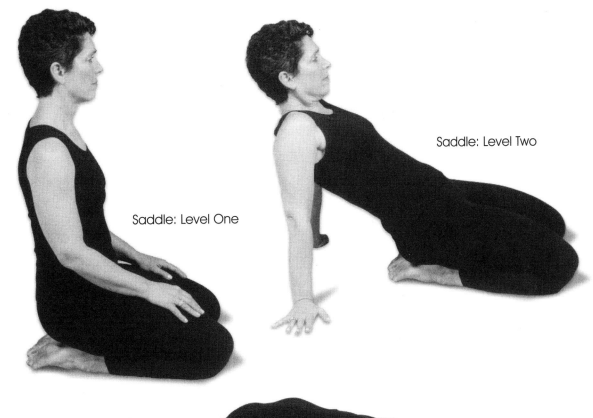

Saddle: Level One

Saddle: Level Two

Saddle: Level Three

[Saddle]

The Saddle helps to strengthen your back and integrate your spine.

▐ Sit on your heels with your knees 6 to 12 inches apart. If this is all you can do for now, hold this (Level One). If you want to take it to the next level, walk back onto your hands (Level Two). For even more stretch, lower down onto your elbows. In the final pose, the top of your head will be on the floor (Level Three).

▐ Remember the soft edge. That edge will shift quickly in Saddle, so don't rush it.

▐ To come up, push down with your legs and hands and lift your chest.

1 to 3 minutes

Child's Pose

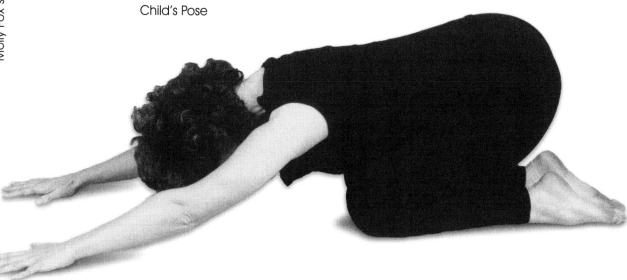

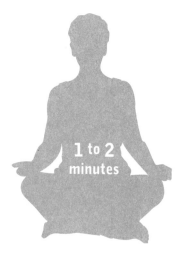

1 to 2 minutes

[**Child's Pose**]

The Child's Pose is a nice gentle release after backbends.

IIII Sit on your heels with your knees 6 inches apart, and bend forward.

IIII Your arms can be forward or back, whichever is more comfortable.

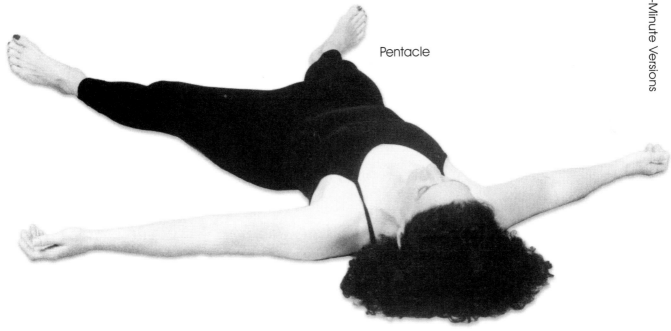

Pentacle

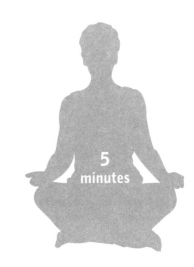

5 minutes

[Pentacle]

▥ Lie on your back with your legs and arms open wide.

▥ Release completely into the floor, relax, and be at peace.

▥ Relax your jaw and throat, and breathe freely.

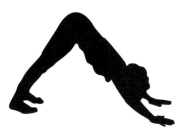

Calming Practice Summary

Becoming calmer—relaxing your nervous system and releasing stress—can be one of the greatest gifts you can give yourself. It will improve your well-being, your outlook on life, and of course support your weight loss goals. Always remember that when you are relaxed and happy you will make choices that support your true intention: joy, health, and peace.

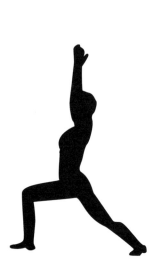

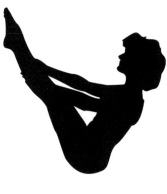

Chapter Seven
Creating a Joyful Practice:
The Basics of Asanas

The real voyage of
discovery consists not
in seeking new land-
scapes but in having
new eyes.

—Marcel Proust

Now that you've had a chance to go through some of the routines and have begun to get familiar with how the poses feel in your body, it's time to look at some details and also at the larger picture.

This chapter will give you many ideas on how to make your yoga weight loss program more enjoyable. The point here is to create a practice of lightness and joy, not one of struggle and effort. You are letting go of something—specifically your weight—but in a more general sense, you're also letting go of many of the things that have been burdening you in your life. You are literally (and figuratively) "lightening up." And when you are light about your yoga practice, you are more likely to show up again and do it tomorrow!

Consistency is everything, and you are far more likely to consistently do something that you love and that brings you joy than to do something that you dread and that ultimately feels like "work." As you follow the various tips and suggestions in this chapter, you will find yourself becoming more and more aware of your body. You will discover the amazing complexity and beauty of your human shape—even at its current weight. You will tap into the power of that body in a new way, and in the process come to love and appreciate it, perhaps for the first time.

Releasing Your Old Tension Patterns

Tension dominates our lives. Through the repetitive nature of our activities, and the constant bombardment of stimuli from our environment, we develop patterns of tension in our bodies as a coping mechanism—a kind of defensive strategy that we need to have just to get by. Some of the physical places in which we "hold" tension are easy to find, feel, and identify. Think of the "knots" in your stomach or gut when you're feeling stressed. Or the tightness in your neck, shoulders, and back. You need to pay particular attention to these areas when you work the asanas.

Upper Back, Shoulders, and Neck

You want your upper back and shoulder area to stay soft—instead of tightening it, take the work of your asanas in your legs and/or arms (depending on what is bearing the weight). As you relax your neck and shoulders, let your collarbones broaden and your upper chest softly lift up. Lauren Davis, owner of Diablo Yoga Center in Danville, California, calls this very top part of your upper chest your "Gorilla Chest." Imagine puffing it up, all the way to your throat.

Another way to release the tension in your upper back is to move your head back. Notice if you jut your chin forward your chest will drop instead of lift. If instead you move your head back from your throat and keep the upward lift of the back of your head, there will be a natural lift of your upper (Gorilla) chest.

Some of what I call the "holding places"—locations in the body where you hold your tension—are less apparent and need careful observation to identify and feel them. Some are unique to you; remember, we are all different—even in the way we hold tension in our bodies. As you progress through your yoga practice you will develop your sensitivity to these "holding places." Notice what happens when you release them. Invariably, when you release tension in one part of your body, some other part of your body will have to do the work.

Feet

One sneaky "holding place" is the feet. When you take your shoes off and step on your yoga mat, begin to be aware of your feet. Are they tight? Drawn up? Can you spread your feet across your mat as if you're spreading peanut butter on a piece of toast? Do your toes stretch away from each other?

You release tension from your feet by slowly and naturally allowing your feet to take your weight. Create a sinking or rooting sensation from your feet into the earth. This action will reconnect you with the natural world. And as much as we try to create a separation from that natural world in the course of our daily lives, that separation remains an illusion.

Legs

When we identify and release our chronic "holding places," we can begin to direct our energy away from these tension spots and toward the parts of our bodies that are meant to work and hold us up. For the most part that will be our legs. When we are bearing weight on our feet, our legs become the workhorses for the poses; when we are bearing weight on our hands, the workhorses will be our arms. When the limbs are working, the torso and the diaphragm can function without gripping up. I've often noticed that beginners in a yoga practice are unconsciously nervous about the new sensations of muscles working. As a result, they will grip up in the shoulders, belly, and other "usual suspects" for tension. When we do this, we are not allowing our legs to fully bear the weight. Remember that the majority of our muscles are in our legs and buttocks. Therein lies our strength. Our legs are meant to be strong and dynamic. Let them shake, rattle, and roll all they want!

Don't be afraid of your legs. They will hold you up and will not let you down.

Diaphragm

Another area where we hold tension is deep in our breathing diaphragm. Stress and the tension of life can lead us to hold our breath or at least to breathe with very shallow breaths. Have you ever observed your own breathing during moments of great tension? Your breaths become short and very shallow. (One reason someone always tells you to "take a deep breath" when you're highly tense and stressed is that deep breathing is incompatible with anxiety.) When you hold your breath, you are not using your very muscular diaphragm muscle, the main muscle used in breathing. This leads to lack of tone not only in the diaphragm but also in the abdominal area and back. When the breath is shortened, your internal organs are not massaged and toned very well. Your diaphragm muscle functions as a pump that works on your internal organs as it expands and contracts. This contributes to the health of your organs.

What to do to release the tension in this part of the body? Well, your diaphragm connects to your rib cage along the whole bottom rim. As you become aware of tension there, mentally relax it and allow the entire circumference of your ribs to expand as you inhale. You will then experience a release of the gripping feeling in your belly at the same time as you feel the expansion of your ribs. Sometimes chronic tension in your belly is related to breathing in a shallow way, to failing to take deep, nourishing breaths that fill the lungs, raise the chest, and expand the ribs. So unravel your tension—reveal the depth of your breath.

Another by-product of releasing your diaphragm is that your pelvic floor and groin will relax and release. By letting your breath descend down to your pelvic floor, you will release chronically held tension in that part of your body. If your pelvic floor is released, you will be able to drop your weight into your legs and feet.

Another place where many people hold tension is the throat and jaw. Take a look to see if this is true for you. Allow your tongue to hang heavy in your mouth; drop your jaw and allow your eyes to get soft. Deep diaphragm breathing will have an effect on your jaw and throat as well.

After spending some time identifying your personal "holding places," explore the softness of your poses. What other muscles have been neglected? Which ones haven't had the opportunity to work because the "holding places" have been overworking? Noticing is the beginning of making change. (Later in the book you will see that noticing, or observing, is the also the first step in changing your eating patterns—see Three Steps Toward Fat-Melting Success in Chapter 13.)

Now that your awareness has expanded, let's begin to learn new ways of working that will target your larger muscles, increase your strength, and accelerate your weight loss.

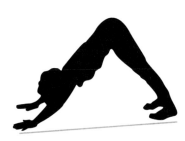

Unravel your tension— reveal the depth of your breath.

Create a Strong Foundation

Creating a strong foundation for your yoga pose is similar to creating a strong foundation when building a house. A house without a strong foundation will tumble or lean or otherwise be uninhabitable. A yoga pose without a solid base will take more effort, be less balanced, and usually create a lot of tension in places where you don't want it, like your neck, back, and shoulders. Using your foundation will also help you burn more calories because you are using your larger muscle groups—your legs and buttocks. That's good news!

So what is your foundation? It is that which touches the earth. The part of your body that touches the earth can use the earth to create a force from which to move. If this seems hard to understand right now, bear with me. It will all become clear soon enough.

The Four Corners: Hands and Feet First

Your hands and feet are your most important foundational body parts. Imagine your favorite dog or cat moving through the world, running or exploring in a field or stalking a bird or squirrel in your backyard. Notice how the animal uses its paws to maneuver through its world. We use our "paws"—our hands and feet—in a similar way when doing our yoga poses.

Your hands can be seen as having "four corners." So can your feet. These four corners can be considered the foundation of any yoga pose. They will be explained in more detail in the paragraphs below. Optimally, we want to balance the weight of the body among the four corners of the hands (when they are supporting weight) and/or the four corners of the feet (when they are supporting weight).

Your Feet

The four corners of your feet are the inner and outer ball and the inner and outer heel. When the weight is evenly distributed among these four corners, the arches lift and the work of the pose is balanced up your leg and into your pelvis. This will get your leg and buttock muscles working more evenly. As you practice your poses, get to know your feet and experience where you naturally place your weight. When your weight goes more to your inner foot, the work will be felt more in the inner thigh and groin and will help your leg turn in. Conversely, when your weight shifts more to the outside foot, your leg will turn out slightly more. Once again, it's all about balance. We are looking for even weight on all four corners.

▥ Distribute your body weight among the four corners of your feet—the inner and outer ball and inner and outer heel of each foot.

▥ Experiment with the strength of your feet by raising all 10 toes up off of the floor. Notice how the arches of your feet lift and your legs feel more muscular and strong.

We get our stability and strength from the foundation of our bodies, particularly our feet and legs. This strength resonates up to a central point—your center—which helps with your balance and creates a sense of connectedness both to the earth and to your own internal power.

Your Hands

In some poses, the hands are part of our foundation. (For example, Downward Facing Dog, page 51). Just as you distributed the weight of your body to the four corners of your feet, on these poses you want to distribute your weight to the four corners of your hand. On your hands the four corners are the index finger and pinky palm knuckle and the inner and outer heel of your hand. Balancing the weight on these four corners is not as easy or natural as it sounds. As we evolved from our primate ancestors, we became an upright species, no longer walking (and bearing weight) on our hands. Yet using them in this way can create strength in the upper body and improve body awareness.

Yes, you can get toned and shapely arms and shoulders from using your hands and arms correctly. When you put weight on the inner part of your hands it affects the inner part of your arm and shoulder; when you put weight on the outer part of your hand it affects the outer part of your arm and shoulder.

▥ Distribute your body weight among the four corners of your hand: the index and pinky finger palm knuckle and the inner and outer lower palm.

▥ Press down on the upper portion of your hand (the index and pinky finger palm knuckle) to take the weight off your wrist. Notice how the underbelly of each arm gets firm, and your shoulders feel more stable.

Just as we want to find a balance of weight among the four corners of our hands or feet, we also want to balance our muscular energy or strength with our bone energy or expansion. Your body works as a unit at all times. There is a general pulsation of energy that moves in and out of your body. Your muscles pull energy and your bones create extension. The following experiment illustrates how powerful the balance between these two forces can be. It will demonstrate to you just how much stronger and more stable we are when we balance our muscle strength with our bone extension. You can feel this by doing it yourself, but you'll really get the idea if you get a friend to assist you.

Extend your arm out to the side in line with your shoulder. First "make a muscle" in your arm with so much effort that you feel your arm bone suck into the shoulder socket. How strong do you feel? If you have a friend near you, ask him to press down on your arm to test your strength. You will probably find that your arm goes down somewhat easily. Now "make a muscle" in your arm and then extend your arm bone out from your chest. Have your friend test your arm again. Notice how much stronger and more stable you are. This little experiment is a great way to experience the balance of muscle and bone energy. When you apply this concept to your poses, you will be amazed at how much more capable you feel and how much easier your poses become. This dynamic energy is what we want to experience in our poses. The pulling-in motion and the stretching-out motion that you did with your arm is what you eventually want to do with all parts of your body. You will wind up creating more energy, getting deeper and stronger in your poses, and of course, burning more calories.

In the previous sections I've made a great number of references to the concept of "foot to pelvic core strength." To access this strength:

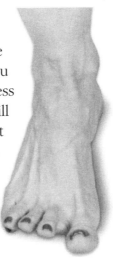

Feet

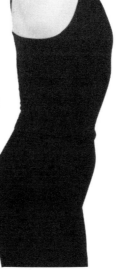

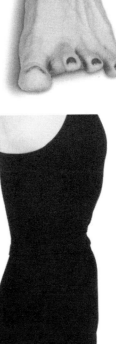

Neutral Pelvis   Hyper-Arched Pelvis

IIII Balance your weight evenly on the four corners of your feet; inner and outer ball and inner and outer heel (see page 163).

IIII Draw strong muscle energy up and into your lower belly or the core of your pelvis. This action is like a hug of your bones by your muscles. The result in your pelvic core will be a straight line from the top of your buttocks in the back, to 2 inches above your pubic bone in front. This is called Neutral Pelvis.

IIII You will balance this drawing up with pressing down and out through the bones of your legs through your feet. This will give you the feeling of steady expansion on the face of the earth.

A Balanced Pelvis

When your pelvis is aligned you stand more securely on your legs and your poses become lighter and more efficient. When this occurs you are able to do more; you will burn more calories with less stress and increased ease. A Balanced Pelvis is a dance of two things:

IIII Moving the top of your leg bones and your groin back to open your pelvic floor and separate your sitting bones; and

IIII Scooping your tailbone under to lengthen your spine and initiate a scoop of your lower belly.

Because of the way that the legs are situated in your pelvis, when you revolve your legs in and back, you increase the natural curve in your lower back. This is a great thing. Most of us spend so much time sitting that we have begun to lose this important curve. This spinal curve is the key to sitting up straight. You will feel your sacrum (a triangular-shaped bone between the tops of your buttocks) move up and in. You will feel your sitting bones move apart. You will feel like your behind is "blossoming" (like a spring bouquet perhaps?). Once your legs are revolved back and your sitting bones open, then you can scoop your tailbone under. This will elongate your spine. This is the dance of the pelvis. Balancing your pelvis in this way is like opening the garage door before driving the car in. Just think what a mess you'd make if you drove the car into the garage before you opened the door. Ouch!

Here are the steps to balance your pelvis:

IIII Take your weight to the inside of your feet. Press down. Draw the muscles of your legs in and up to your pelvis. "Make a muscle" with (i.e., contract) your legs. Feel as if you are creating tone and shape.

▥ Keeping your muscles firm, revolve your legs inward so that the top of your legs and inner thighs move back and open wide, creating space between your sitting bones.

▥ Once the "garage door has opened," scoop your tailbone under into the free space. Feel a strong lift up from your lower belly.

▥ As you scoop your tailbone under, extend that bone extension down and out through your legs. You will feel your buttock flesh sweep down and around your pelvis, creating a firmness and stability for your pelvis.

This balance of drawing in and out will be like a pulsation. You can use the visual image of a tree: as a tree starts to grow from a seed, it first creates the roots it needs for stability; then, from that same seed, it grows leaves, fruit, and branches.

This same concept applies to your hands and the center of your heart or chest, especially when you are bearing weight on your hands. The weight is evenly spread through your hands in Downward Facing Dog (page 51). From the firm foundation of your hands you draw strong muscle energy up to your heart center (the center of your chest). This action will make your chest expand, your collarbones broaden and lift, and your shoulders draw flat on your back and down (see photo).

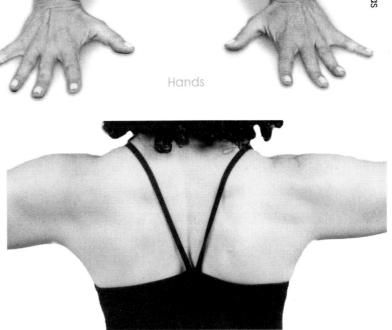

Hands

Shoulder Blades on Your Back

Miscellaneous Tips

The following tips should be considered refinements. They will help you align your body in such a way that you will experience more freedom and ease. Don't even worry about these until you are comfortable with the basic postures. Once you are, consider using each of these as a daily focus to improve your pose. For example, on one day, concentrate on extending out at the top of your head. Use these tips, which will help you access your muscular power and your innate grace, to create some deeper awareness from which to honor your body and your self. Enjoy!

- When moving your feet or hands or when coming up from a forward bend, push down to come up.
- Extend out and up from the crown of your head.
- Think of moving the soft palate in your mouth back and up like you are practicing an inner smile; this will align your head over the central axis of your body. (You can find your soft palate by running your tongue across the hard palate, which is the hard part of the roof of your mouth. Just behind that is your soft palate.)
- Remember that your inner thighs move back and in and your tailbone tucks under. This is a dance, and one aspect of it should not overpower the other. The dance is achieved by balancing the muscular strength and the expansive pressing down and out.

Work at Your EDGE, Not Beyond or Before

Your EDGE is the place that is a balance of "doing" and "being." It is the dance of strong and stable with soft and easy. Be aware that your mind often gives up before your body. I like to use the example of wasabi on sushi. When you eat sushi for the first time, you only put a touch of wasabi on your sushi. As you eat it more often you add more—or you decide not to use it at all. You adapt. You develop your taste preferences (how much of it you like, or if you don't like it at all). The same will happen with your mind and your yoga practice: You can tailor the program to your personal needs, which is entirely in keeping with the whole spirit of this program, both the asana practice and the eating plan. Here are some guidelines to help you find your personal intensity EDGE:

- Your inhale and exhale are for the most part free and even.
- Your muscles may quiver, shake, and ache, yet you can stay calm.

▥ You experience a sense of calm in the presence of dynamic activity, like being in the eye of the hurricane.

Remember, when exploring your own intensity EDGE as well as when doing any of the practices, take breaks as needed. When you have recovered—that is, when the intensity has been brought down—start again where you left off. The Child's Pose (which I like to call the Progressive Adult Pose, see Chapter 4) is well suited to this purpose.

Aligning Your Attitude

Aligning your body, mind, and spirit with your goal is key to a happy experience. In the weight loss journey, one of the frequent obstacles encountered by many dieters is that they lose sight of their purpose and goal; their mind and spirit are not aligned with that goal and are resisting it, resulting in lost motivation, resentment, and feelings of denial. You need to realign your body, mind, and spirit to your vision, whether it be for a better body or a happier, fuller life (or both!). Aligning your body is critical, so that your movements are efficient and yet sufficiently stressful to the muscles to create the result you want: strong muscles and loss of inches and fat. When your body is aligned, your muscles will develop evenly. You may experience more freedom and lightness in your pose. It will also allow your energy to move freely through your body and give you a sense of balancing on your bones. When your body is aligned, your spine for the most part returns to its natural curves and your legs and arms will do the work, so your torso can be free to receive and deliver your breath.

It is not just your body that practices yoga better when it is aligned properly. So do your mind and heart. The word "anusara" means to flow with divine grace, and Anusara yoga is a system of hatha yoga designed by John Friend. According to Friend, "A pure attitude during the performance of an asana purifies the body and mind, and lets the light of the heart freely shine out."

This alignment with your innate goodness and the fullness of your potential—abilities within you that are both manifested and unmanifested—will bring joy and pleasure to your practice and help keep you from practicing with unnecessary tension. Take a moment to go inside yourself and create a personal spiritual reference point that brings about this heart-based connection.

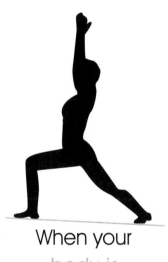

When your body is aligned, your muscles will develop evenly.

Celebrate Your Pose!

Every time you strike a pose you have the opportunity to celebrate yourself. My coach, Judy Talesnick, says that when she takes a pose she begins with affirmations like "Yeah, me!," "I am fit and getting fitter," and "I am beautiful and getting more beautiful every day." This is your opportunity to change your internal voice. Cut off that negativity at the pass. Your mind can only think of one thing at a time—so have it think of something positive. Some examples of positive self-talk might be "You go, girl" or "I am strong, beautiful, and thin, and getting thinner every day." Let your heart get connected to your poses. Lift your heart to the sky and connect with your higher self, that part of you that is whole and complete. Find your connection to something bigger, something beautiful, something that is nature itself.

Because ultimately, that is who you are.

Do Something Every Day

It takes time to develop new habits. We have found that people who have created new activity habits are more likely to continue being active. Even if you can only practice 5 or 10 minutes one day, do it anyway. How much you do is not as important as the fact that you do it, and that you do it consistently. Doing it will keep you positive and will condition your mind to expect a successful experience. That continued conditioning will keep you from giving up. You may feel like just "going with the flow" one day and not practicing because you don't feel like it. Be bigger than just your momentary feelings. Notice them, honor them, but be willing to look at other solutions. If you are very tired, for example, try the Energy Practice or the Calming Practice. The solutions can be different depending on who you are.

Make Changes over Time

The success of any program is found in consistency—do something with regularity over a period of time, and you have a recipe for success. If you look at this as a long-range commitment, it will be easier to adapt these changes into your life in a way that will be easy, effortless, and effective. Think long term—it's what you do 90 percent of the time that counts. If, for example, we recommend that you do something every day, and for one day or two days you don't, just start again. Know that it is the focus on the larger picture that creates success. Beating yourself up for being human and having a life never works.

It may be helpful to realign yourself with your spiritual nature when you don't accomplish your "to-do list." Put a positive spin on it. For example, suppose you didn't have time to practice one day because you needed to take your daughter to school for Parent-Teacher Day. Acknowledge yourself as the type of person who has her priorities in order. There is always a way to take a "higher spin" on what could have been an opportunity to beat yourself up. Try it. It really works.

In summary:

- Become aware of chronic tensions and learn how to release them.
- Start waking up your body to new possibilities.
- Develop the strength of your legs which will, in turn, allow your breath to be free. (If you aren't using the strength of your legs when holding a pose, you're probably holding your breath).
- Use your EDGE to develop your strength and flexibility over time. (Remember that working at your EDGE will make you push yourself just enough so that you get stronger and burn more calories and start losing weight; get familiar with your EDGE so you know when not to give up!)
- Find the joy and the freedom in each pose.
- Open the door to allow you to love yourself exactly the way you are.

When in doubt, enjoy the fact that you are healthy and breathing and have the opportunity to do this practice.

And never forget to check in on your inner smile.

Chapter Eight
Breath, Meditation, and Mindfulness

Joy is within.
Meditate.

—Swami Muktananda

The practice of mindfulness—being conscious of your thoughts, feelings, and sensations—is key to weight loss. Mindfulness is a Buddhist principle. According to Jon Kabat-Zinn, author of *Wherever You Go, There You Are,* mindfulness is defined as "paying attention in a particular way: on purpose, in the present moment, and nonjudgmentally." He goes on to say, "This kind of attention nurtures greater awareness, clarity and acceptance of present-moment reality. It wakes us up to the fact that our lives unfold only in moments." Finally, he concludes, "If we are not fully present for many of those moments, we may not only miss what is most valuable in our lives but also fail to realize the richness and the depth of our possibilities for growth and transformation."

We are overweight for a reason. No matter how many times we go on a diet and exercise program, we will not be truly successful until we uncover the reasons that we overeat in the first place, and address them honestly, openly, and without fear. For many of us the question comes down to this: What are the feelings that we don't want to feel?

Consider my own personal experience with feelings and weight loss. Having grown up in the 99th percentile of height and weight, I always had the experience of being just plain big. That number must have made a real impression on me, because I remember always being aware of the fact that only 1 percent of the population was bigger than I. This was not good news. Layered upon that knowledge was the feeling I had that big girls were not feminine or pretty. I was good at sports, dance, and most things physical, but I just wanted to look thin and waiflike in a bathing suit.

As I grew up, I found lots of ways to not feel those feelings of inadequacy. I tried every diet available. I began to exercise—first a little, then a lot, then obsessively just to maintain my weight. The exercise itself was obviously not a bad thing, but I wasn't doing it for healthy reasons. It turned into a punishment for being the wrong size, and not a delicious activity to help me enjoy my body. And how many times did I exercise hard just to punish myself for overeating? I remember one time hating myself so much for having a piece of cake at dinner that I went out almost immediately for a grueling five-mile run.

There's a name for this kind of obsessive exercising, motivated only by a desire to burn up calories. It's called exercise bulimia. I was doing everything except uncovering the reasons that I was overeating in the first place. I was doing everything possible to avoid the feeling that I was so afraid to feel—the feeling of being big, bad, and different. I began the process of mindful meditation. And through that process, I was able to allow the feelings to unfold and, finally, the tears underneath to flow.

I cried for a long time. I gave myself permission to cry for as long as I needed to. I will never forget the day that I realized I did not have to be afraid of my tears and my feelings and that the tears wouldn't last forever. I knew that if I could just give myself permission to feel what I was feeling, at some point I would stop crying. Through the process of allowing myself to both discover and uncover my deepest fears and feelings, I came to accept my body as it is and to learn and embrace the things that I need to do to stay healthy and fit. I exercise a moderate amount. I practice yoga regularly. I lift weights twice a week and love it passionately.

I do a process I call "feeling upkeep," a kind of emotional tune-up. When feelings come up for me, even if they're uncomfortable, I give myself complete permission to feel them. If I need to lie down and cry for a while, guess what? That's just what I do. I let it out and get on with life. I've discovered that I have to fully give in to the feelings, without holding back. I am totally present to them. And by releasing the fear of my feelings, they have become my greatest ally.

I invite you to know yourself and your feelings. Embrace them and experience them fully. After all, they are yours and no one else's—no one ever can take them from you and no one feels them exactly the way you do. They are unique to you, and you deserve to

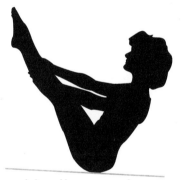

I invite you to know yourself and your feelings.

feel them fully. And at the other end is the pure joy of your beauty, grace, and divine spirit.

You can be mindful of your feelings all day long. Experience your sadness, your anger, your fear, and your joy. (This does not mean you should give yourself permission to go on a "rage attack" when you are angry; it just means that you need to get in touch with what you are feeling so that you can confront that feeling honestly rather than stifle it, ignore it, push it down, or deny it.) There are many more productive ways to express your anger besides laying out the poor guy that cuts you off on the freeway. My preferred way is to take a plastic bat and bash my bed. This is a fantastic technique used in a phenomenal personal development program called the Hoffman Quadrinity Process. I have found by doing it that I have let go of a lot of old anger.

Since I became more in touch with my feelings, I have also found myself expressing my joy a lot more. As a kid I was super happy and outrageously inquisitive. But I grew up feeling like it was "just too much." As one of our teachers back in the days of the Actors Institute used to say, "Somebody told you to keep it down one too many times!" I learned to squelch my joy and passions. But through mindful meditation I have come to learn how to surround myself with people who support my sense of fun and love of life. I no longer have to "keep it down."

Thanks to the process of welcoming my feelings and letting them out to be expressed in appropriate ways, I find myself eating less for emotional reasons and more because I am hungry. I still love a good chocolate chip cookie now and then—but I love it for how it tastes and feels in my mouth, and I'm able to control how much I'll indulge. I'm no longer using the cookie to take away my pain.

In the following sections, we'll show you some wonderful techniques for developing breathing and meditation practices that will enhance your ability to lose weight by helping you to increase mindfulness and consciousness. These are two powerful tools to help you discover what led you to gain the weight in the first place.

Getting Ready for Breathing Practices

Oxygen is more important to being alive than food or water. Obviously if we stopped breathing, we would die; we can go much longer without food or water than we can without air. It is also true that we don't have to think about breathing; it happens automatically. Good thing for us! But did you know that the respiratory system is the one system that is both involuntary and voluntary? You can affect your breath with your mind and your thoughts, just as your thoughts affect your breathing patterns—even subconsciously. When we become nervous, excited, anxious, or face stress, the breath shortens. We either hold our breath or take shallow breaths, most of the time without even thinking about it. Conversely, when we are in love or are playing with a baby or a puppy, our breath may slow down and become more even. We breathe deeper, almost automatically. So our unconscious thoughts profoundly influence our breath, just as our conscious thoughts do.

Just by paying attention, we can change the quality of our breath. Why is this a good thing? Because consciously slowing down or deepening your breath helps to balance your nervous system.

The breathing practices that follow will accomplish the above and ultimately bring down chronic levels of stress. They can give you the energy to engage in a dynamic life.

Basic Tips on Breathing Practice

Everybody breathes. So what's the big deal? Why do we need special breathing practices, anyway?

Although breath is synonymous with life and everybody does it, consciously developing your breathing muscles and freeing up your breath by releasing restrictions is like Alice opening up the door to Wonderland. You will find there a magical pathway to your own inner life that will create health, well-being, and inner peace. And when you have that as a foundation, weight loss will become effortless.

- Breathe in and out through your nose unless stated otherwise. This helps to filter the air and slows down the breathing process so that it becomes more meditative.
- Find your own rhythm. Your rhythm is where the inhale and exhale are even and there is no stress or sense of pulling or pushing. You want ease and consistency. If you feel tensions, stop, slow down, and relax your jaw, your body, and your mind.
- Sit up tall with a straight spine. You can sit in an easy sitting pose on a blanket, against a wall, or in a chair with your feet on the floor.

Breathing with an Open Heart

I have noticed that my Breathing Practice takes on different qualities depending on my attitude. If I approach my breathing practice determined to control it, with lots of "should dos" and "must dos" floating around in my head, it is never particularly pleasurable and I lose the wonderful sense of connecting to spirit. But if I practice with an open heart, if I let myself feel the inner and outer connections of my breath with the universe, the whole experience changes and I become lighter.

Ways of Practicing with an Attitude of Openheartedness

Create a feeling—and a physical sensation—of love; then imagine yourself breathing that in with each breath. This image will impart a lightness and a sweetness to your whole body.

Basic Easy Breath

Breathe in and out through your nose. As you inhale, imagine drawing your breath up and in through your collarbones. (Although this is not physically possible, it works as a nice metaphor to maximize your breath.) As you take air in, feel your lungs fill up, your chest expand, and finally, your belly move. Then, when you exhale, keep the natural lift of your heart as your breath first leaves your belly then travels up. Keep your inhale and your exhale even. A good way to practice is "four counts inhale," "four counts exhale." Gradually extend the length of time so that the nice even breaths get longer and slower. Observe the spaces between your breath without tension.

Bellows Breath

Take a full deep breath, in and out. Then inhale half of a breath while creating a lift of your rib cage. Make sharp exhalations through your nose, initiated by pumping your lowest belly muscles up, back, and in. This is like stoking your own inner fire with your bellows. At first you may snort, spit, and generally not be too smooth. That's fine. Your breathing will deepen and become smoother with practice. Start off slow and deep. Change the rhythm. See how it feels.

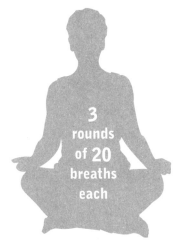

3 rounds of 20 breaths each

Deep Sea Breath

You may remember this breathing practice from our discussion of it in Chapter 4. I recommend that you do it for both your Energy Practice and Strength Practice.

Breathe in and out through your nose while slightly constricting the back of your throat. It will feel like you are breathing through your throat. A good way to practice this is to inhale a breath and exhale the sound of "Ahhhhhhhh" out of your mouth. Next breathe in, and close your mouth as you make the "Ahhhhhhh" sound in your throat. The beauty of this breathing practice is that the feel and sound of your breath actually assists in its meditative qualities. By keeping your attention on the quality of your Deep Sea Breath during your asana practice, you will be aware of when you are pushing too hard and need to back off, or when your mood is wandering and you need to kick up your intensity.

Meditation is the natural counterpart to breathing. There is no one "right" way to do meditation. Many people are initially put off by the fact that they believe meditation is very complicated, and it is going to be difficult to learn, or require that they have some special abilities to "put themselves in a trance." A lot of beginners are worried that they can't "turn off their thoughts." Truth is, you don't have to (and probably won't be able to in the beginning anyway).

Don't worry about it. Meditation can be as simple as sitting quietly and concentrating on your breath. If mundane thoughts about things like picking up the dry cleaning, or planning what to eat for dinner, intrude—and it's inevitable that they will—just keep returning to what you are focused on. It's all good.

The meditation practices that follow are meant to give you some ideas about how to get started. Once you do, you will wonder how you ever lived without it.

Meditation Practice

The process of slowing down and freeing up your breath that we spoke about in the last section can result in the desire to go "inside" and spend some time in the world behind your eyes. Meditation is an opportunity to get to know your thoughts, to really experience them. It is a practice that brings you home to you.

As you will learn in Chapter 12, most eating is unconscious. The result of that unconsciousness is that we wind up acquiring habits that are counterproductive and not in alignment with our goals. We eat emotionally, we eat because we're stressed, or we eat compulsively almost without conscious awareness of what (and how much) we are consuming. None of these eating styles and patterns is conducive to weight loss, let alone to a healthy relationship with food or a positive attitude about nourishing our bodies. Meditation is a terrific way to slow down, regroup, and consider what we really want out of life. It's a way to connect with your less frantic self, to experience your body and appreciate its need for good wholesome nourishment, and ultimately to develop the kind of self-love that will serve you so well in your weight loss journey.

In the daily process of living our lives, most of us get caught up in what we are doing, who we think we are, and how we present that to the world. We carry around plenty of guilt about the past and concerns about the future. This leaves no time for what I call the "Perfect Present." Rarely do we slow down enough to experience the "Now," to be, as they say, "in the moment."

Meditation allows us to spend time observing the space between our thoughts. It allows us to observe them without getting attached to them; it allows us to experience the all-so-infrequent quiet in the midst of the constant chatter in our minds. That space is where we can make contact with our Essence—with who we really are. It is in that quiet space that we can feel the Universal Energy that connects us all, that emanates from our hearts, and is a personal and unique— yet profoundly ordinary—experience.

When they first begin a meditation practice, many people think that they have to "turn off" their thoughts, and find that very difficult to do. Actually, according to Jon Kabat-Zinn, meditation is not the absence of thoughts, but the awareness of thoughts, and of course, awareness of the quiet space between them. Don't feel you have to "turn off" the chatter in your mind; at first that will be next to impossible to do anyway. Simply experience the thoughts. Imagine them floating in the clouds.

I mentioned earlier the concept of not getting "attached" to thoughts. A good example of that is Jonny's experience when he stopped smoking some 20 years ago. He would still have the thought that he would like a cigarette—but he didn't have to do anything about it. He wouldn't empower it by reaching for the pack. Instead, he just noticed it floating by and thought to himself, "Hmm, that's interesting, there goes that thought that it would be nice to have a cigarette." That's what I mean by not getting attached.

The thoughts you notice floating by during your meditation can range from the trivial ("I have to return that overdue video!") to the

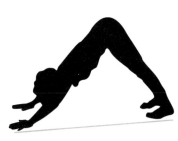

Meditation **allows us to spend time observing the space between our thoughts.**

disturbing ("I'll never amount to anything," "I'll never lose weight," "This meditation thing sucks"). But just because you notice them doesn't mean you have to attach any power or mass to them. Instead, just observe them floating by and go back to connecting with your breath. In Buddhist philosophy this is referred to as "Beginner's mind" or "becoming the observer." That's what we want to do in meditation. It is a practice of getting to know "what's so."

This is how you begin to connect with your own personal truth. You can't do it wrong. Just look at what's there. Notice it, and move on.

Here's how you get started. Go to your sacred personal space. Shut the door and set up the area so you will not be disturbed. Sit tall with an erect spine just as you would in a Breathing Practice.

Start this practice with a short amount of time (5 minutes) and build up; it's better to do a short amount of time consistently than to do a longer time infrequently and sporadically. Sometimes it is helpful to journal after your meditation so that you can become more aware of your inner thoughts and patterns.

Enjoy!

Basic Breathing Meditation

Sit comfortably. Bring your attention and awareness to your breath. Feel the inhale, the exhale, and the spaces between. Expand your awareness to include the physical sensations in your body as you breathe. Feel your chest expand, the gentle movement of your belly, and the sensation in your throat. As your mind wanders and various thoughts float by in your consciousness, redirect your attention to your breath. You may try saying to yourself "Thinking" when you are thinking and "Breathing" when you are breathing to assist in heightening your awareness of what is so.

Breathing Love Meditation

Again, sit comfortably. Bring your attention to your breathing. As you breathe in, think to yourself the word "love." Feel like you're breathing in the essence of love. As you breathe out, repeat the process. Let love surround you. In your mind's eye you can envision someone you love and stoke the "love fire." If there isn't anyone like that in your life right now, that's fine. You can still experience how this feeling of love is generated from you. It's your own ability to love. Send this love from you to you. Bathe in the sweetness of it.

Perhaps you can even send this love to someone with whom you are struggling. Here you can really feel the effects of forgiveness. By sending love to a rival you let go of all the negative thoughts and energy that really affect only you in the end. You may not completely release your anger or upset, but you will have created the beginnings of forgiveness.

After meditation, observe how you feel. How does it feel to love yourself? Or even to love your rival?

Walking Meditation

Here's an interesting variation for you: Try walking during your meditation practice. Before you set out, commit to the idea that this walk is going to be a meditative practice. It's not about window shopping. Rather, you're bringing your meditative "headset" into the open air.

You will want to choose a focus. Some suggestions:

- Focus on your breath. Find a comfortable length for your inhale and exhale. Then pace your strides to your breath. For example, you might choose four steps for your inhale and four steps for your exhale.
- Focus on a color. You can choose a color to discover during your walk. If you choose green, for example, look for all the places that you see green. See green as often as you can. This observing meditation can be fun and helps to develop our powers of observation. Notice that when you are looking for something, it tends to appear in your universe more often. Are there any ways you can transfer this experience to your life?

I use the above meditation and focus on joy. You'd be surprised how often I see happiness all around me.

Meditating on the Everyday

Beginning a daily meditation practice can significantly improve your life. When I start my day with a seated meditation my whole day takes on a softness, a smoothness that otherwise doesn't exist. I have a daily meditation practice during which I sit with the intention of being still and observing the silence. It is truly one of the sweetest parts of my day. I usually have my two dogs, Max and Grace Kali, on my lap, which makes it extra delicious.

In doing this, I began to observe that I could become more present and mindful during the "everydayness" of life (even while doing the dishes!). Here are some of the ways that I've been able to do that.

Household Chores

Who would ever think that doing the dishes or scrubbing the bathtub could be a meditation? I know it seems like a stretch, but the truth is, it can. Everything depends on your attitude and perspective. It can be any way you want it to be. Every moment of every day we can choose to approach our activities in the way that is most empowering. The more open you are, the more you will become aware of just how much is available to you at all times. You will begin to see how much the Universe offers on any given day at any given moment. You will find that there are outrageous gifts just waiting for you to pluck them up and experience them with delight.

When scrubbing the tub or doing the dishes, slow down. See the tub. See the dish. Observe the food on the dishes, and the soap as it starts to foam. See the process of cleaning unfold before your eyes. See it through the eyes of a child eager to play and to contribute. Your life is better when your dishes are done and your tub is clean—why not choose to enjoy giving yourself that gift?

Gardening

I don't have a large garden. My gardening experience was limited to years of living in New York City, where the best I was able to do was to become a potted-plant gardener with only the lightest of green thumbs. But I did enjoy what I did. Gardening became a wonderful "present moment" in which I could slow down and take in what was happening around me. While you garden, dig in the dirt like you did when you were a kid. Pick flowers that you enjoy; you know the colors and smells that make you feel good. And when you are out in your garden—even if your garden is a few potted plants and herbs—observe the colors, the textures, the scents, and the magnificence of nature. It's there in a potted plant just as surely as it's in an award-winning greenhouse!

This magnificence is reflected back to you, as you are a force of nature as well.

Spend Time with Children and Animals

Have you ever noticed that when you see a small puppy or baby, you immediately break out into a big smile? This inner joy that bubbles up is our true natural essence. Take advantage of how we are naturally wired. When you are out in the world and see a baby or any little sentient being that you enjoy being with, stop! Take the time to enjoy the experience. Say hi to the baby, or stop and pet the animal. (Asking first, of course, would be a good idea! But almost no one will say "no.")

Help yourself to nature's greatest gift: itself.

Take a Bubble Bath

Partake in a pleasure practice. Soaking in a tub can be a sensual, delicious way to enjoy your body and the thousands of nerve endings you have in it. Prepare the bath as if you're making a beautiful setting for a lover. Take the time you would take for him or her. Light some candles, play some music, get the atmosphere just right. Choose bubbles or aromatherapy oils. Make the choices that will create the most pleasure for you.

You may need to experiment a bit to discover what it is you really do enjoy. It may have been a long time since you checked in with yourself to see what it is that you truly desire, to see what turns you on and makes you smile. Meditate on the sensual experience. Really experience the physical sensations, the smells, the texture and temperature of the water—the whole experience.

These are just a few of the ways you can practice your natural meditative abilities in everyday settings. With practice, you can really learn to enjoy your daily tasks. Meditate on the mundane . . . and it will become magic!

Ultimately, nothing takes the place of doing a sitting meditation every morning. Such a daily practice creates a strong foundation for self-care. Accept and love your body and you will create the possibility to transform it into almost anything you can imagine.

Chapter Nine
Two-Week Sample Practice

Twenty years from now you
will be more disappointed
by the things you didn't do
than by the ones you did.
So throw off the bowlines.
Sail away from the safe
harbor. Catch the trade
winds in your sails.
Explore. Dream. Discover.

—Mark Twain

Although there is no perfect way for any one person to practice, I would like to offer samples of how you might put together a personal yoga practice for yourself. You can adapt these practices in any way that works for you, whether you have 20 minutes available or just 10. For example, if you only have 10 minutes, just do one of the Flow practices, such as the Bridge Flow.

A good rule of thumb is to do less more consistently as opposed to doing a lot every once in a while. Whatever you do, enjoy it, and do it for yourself. If you fall short of what you think you should do, let it go and take some kind of action. Maybe the Sun Salutation is just what you need.

Here are some suggestions to consider when planning your weekly practice schedule.

- If on any given day you are really tired, do the Calming Practice.
- If you lack energy, practice the Energy routine.

▥ If you want to experience your power and want a strong, challenging practice, jump into the Strength routine.

▥ Try splitting up your practice; you can do 20 minutes in the morning and 20 in the evening.

If you have a hard time just getting up and onto your yoga mat, make a deal with yourself: You are only going to do the Mountain Pose. Then say, "Hmmm . . . let's do a Stretch Up and a Forward Bend." Let the natural desire, the organic high, come to you. We are wired to move. Just be open.

Remember that this is just a guide and a sample, much like the two-week eating plan in Chapter 11. Feel free to exchange any of the practices with any of the other practices and make up your own combinations. It's the same thing with the meditations and breathing exercises. I have found that Deep Sea Breath goes more naturally with Strength Practice and the Energy Practice, and Bellows Breath is a great warm-up for your Energy Practice. Easy Breath goes with everything.

Feel free to make your own discoveries about what fits with what. Also allow yourself to extend the time you meditate as you become more comfortable with the practice of meditation. You may start with as few minutes as you like—some people begin their practice with as little as a minute or two a day—but feel free to expand that at your own pace.

Week One

MONDAY	**40-Minute Energy Practice** Bellows Breath Breathing Love Meditation Journal in your food diary
TUESDAY	**40-Minute Strength Practice** Easy Breathing Walking Meditation Journal in your food diary
WEDNESDAY	**20-Minute Energy Practice/20-Minute Calming Practice** Bellows Breath Basic Breathing Meditation Journal in your food diary
THURSDAY	**40-Minute Strength Practice** Breathing with an Open Heart Breathing Love Meditation Journal in your food diary
FRIDAY	**40-Minute Energy Practice** Bellows Breath Scented-oil bath Journal in your food diary
SATURDAY	**20-Minute Strength Practice/20-Minute Calming Practice** Basic Breathing Practice Breathing Love Meditation Journal in your food diary
SUNDAY	**20-Minute Calming Practice** Deep Sea Breath Basic Breathing Meditation Journal in your food diary

Week Two

MONDAY	**20-Minute Energy Practice/20-Minute Strength Practice** Bellows Breath Walking Meditation Journal in your food diary
TUESDAY	**40-Minute Energy Practice** Bellows Breath Breathing Love Meditation Journal in your food diary
WEDNESDAY	**40-Minute Strength Practice** Deep Sea Breath Basic Breathing Meditation Journal in your food diary
THURSDAY	**40-Minute Calming Practice** Breathing with an Open Heart Walking Meditation Journal in your food diary
FRIDAY	**20-Minute Energy Practice /20-Minute Calming Practice** Bellows Breath Breathing Love Meditation Journal in your food diary
SATURDAY	**40-Minute Energy Practice** Bellows Breath Basic Breath Meditation Journal in your food diary
SUNDAY	**Scented-oil bath** Meditation Practice of Your Choice

Part Three
The Yoga Weight Loss Eating Plan

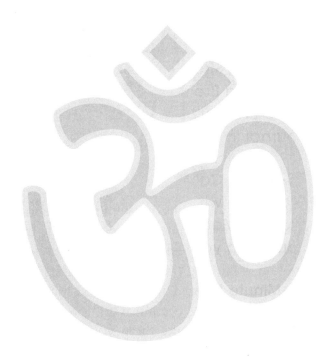

Tell me what you eat, and I will tell you what you are.

—Jean-Anthelme Brillat-Savarin,
French gourmet and author, *The Physiology of Taste*

Chapter Ten
Overview:
The Yoga Weight Loss Philosophy

If we did all the
things we are capable
of doing we would
literally astound
ourselves.

—Thomas Edison

In all our years of counseling people in nutrition and health, one basic truth we've come to respect is this: Everybody's different.

This basic truth encompasses the entirety of the yoga weight loss program, including the exercise sections that precede this part of the book. We hope we have conveyed that what will make Molly Fox's Yoga Weight Loss Program work for you is your willingness to adapt the routines and make them your own. Now we want you to keep that same spirit firmly in mind as you read through the following sections about nutrition and diet.

One day, maybe within the next 10 years, we will know much more about the genetic component of weight gain and loss. Drug companies are developing drugs that interfere with the expression of specific genes that program some of us to gain weight more easily than others, and these genes are different in different people. One day we may well have a pharmacology that is directed specifically to the individual. But right now, in many ways, we are still fumbling. (Several theories of "metabolic typing" have been proposed, but in our opinion none have yet proven themselves to be either accurate enough or practical enough to be adapted for the general public.)

Meanwhile, time and again it is confirmed in our daily practices—and in those of our colleagues around the country—that no single diet works for everyone. Some people clearly do well on high-protein diets, and some people do not. Some people thrive on vegetarian diets (not as many as you might think, by the way), whereas others respond by becoming lackadaisical and tired on a diet without meat. We see on a regular basis how red meat gives some people energy, but we also see how it makes others feel heavy; how milk gives some people gas and bloat and creates mucus, while others seem to be able to drink milk on a daily basis with no problems whatsoever.

Undoubtedly, you have observed the same thing in your own life. Who doesn't have a friend who seems to be able to eat almost anything, from the richest ice cream to the worst fast-food meal, and never put on a pound? And who doesn't know of people who seem to gain weight if they as much as look at fattening foods? (Both of us belong to the latter category!)

Different Strokes for Different Folks

Jonny consulted for a company that delivered gourmet food to the home, specifically for people who needed to be on controlled diets to lose weight. It was an educational experience. When he came on as a consultant, the meals that were being sent out were calorie controlled, but the carbohydrate content was high. Some people were indeed losing weight, but others were not. Those who were not were sure that the high carbohydrate content of the meals was keeping them from losing weight, possibly due to individual metabolic factors such as an inability to process sugar effectively. (Jonny believes that in most cases they were exactly right.)

In response to this feedback, Jonny changed the meal plan to more resemble a "zone-like" diet—a plan based around protein, good fats, and tons of vegetables with a smattering of starches, a program he feels strongly is healthy for most people. The results were interesting. Many people immediately reported feeling less hungry, more satisfied, and less likely to "cheat." These individuals started to see their weight move in a positive direction, at different rates to be sure, but in a positive direction nonetheless.

Interestingly, the people who had fared well on the previous high-carbohydrate plan complained bitterly. They missed the treats that had been included in their meal plan. They missed the pasta and rice in their dishes. They didn't feel satisfied, and their weight loss frequently stopped. Ultimately, Jonny put in place two completely different menus to satisfy both factions.

Truth be told, two plans weren't enough. There are so many individual variations in the way people metabolize and utilize food and calories that virtually every menu—to be ideal—needs to be designed with the specific person who is going to follow it in mind. Obviously this is not possible to do in any book, including this one. We want you to understand this well so that you can make the best use of the following plan. By understanding the spirit of the plan—and the individual variations in response that are likely to occur with any plan— you will be best able, in the spirit of true yoga consciousness, to make it work for you instead of you being a slave to it.

We also know that people learn differently: Some of us are "hands-on" people who learn best by doing; some are "visual," and learn by seeing; and some learn best by listening. Health club salespeople are taught that if their potential member is a "visual" person, she is most likely to benefit from being shown around the club rather than being talked to in the office. If a potential member is a "hands-on" person, he is going to want to hold a brochure in his hands, or have a demonstration of the equipment. And if the potential member is an auditory person, she will respond best to talking and verbal interaction.

It's much the same thing with diets. Some people respond well to a menu of choices rather than a set prescription for eating. Others much prefer the structure of knowing exactly what they can eat, and when. They don't want to have to "think" too much—they just want to follow a simple, laid-out program. The spirit of Molly Fox's Yoga Weight Loss Program is that it leans toward the first choice: We want you to increase your consciousness about food and about your body's relationship to it. We want you to be able to think on your feet—to make intelligent and wise choices about the food that most sustains and nurtures you while serving you in attaining your fitness and weight goals.

But we also recognize that for many people, this increased consciousness and awareness is best achieved gradually, through a more structured program, so we've put together a specific two-week plan that you can follow exactly as written. We hope you will use it as a guide to discovering what works for you and to help you develop your own weight loss program as time goes on.

This plan can be useful to you in a number of ways. For one thing, it is portion controlled. It comes as a huge shock to most people in our culture, who are used to extravagantly oversized restaurant portions, to see what normal portions, such as 4 or 5 ounces of meat or fish, 2 ounces of pasta or cereal, or 1 tablespoon of oil, really look like. This plan will help you become conscious of exactly how much food you really need both to satisfy you and to allow you to steadily lose body fat and weight. It would be a great idea to buy a food scale—it's an ultimate "conscious-raising" tool and you'll learn a heck of a lot about portion size by using it.

The plan also stresses the kinds of foods Jonny believes work best for most people: protein, vegetables, good fats, and reduced starches. When you finish the two-week sample plan, you should be much more able to craft your own meals according to these healthful guidelines, while making the necessary adjustments to accommodate your own individual metabolism.

So, for those of you who need or desire structure in your diet, here is a perfect two-week menu plan that you can follow to the letter. You don't have to think about anything—just follow the instructions and eat the food! However, you also have some options. For one thing, any meal can be substituted for any other meal. If you don't like the lunch on a given day, just use a lunch from another day—or even a breakfast or dinner. And, as you will see from the instructions, you can make the day's menu a little more filling by adding a snack, or a little less so by removing one.

It's also a fact of life that most people today live impossibly busy and complicated lives that frequently include eating out and traveling, so we've come up with some options that allow you to make substitutions that will work just as well as the meals we've given you. Simply use the "customized menu" option at the end of the two-week eating plan (page 228). It allows you to create a meal by choosing from column A, from column B, and from column C. If you like, you can substitute any meal from the "customized menu" for any of the dinners or lunches on the diet.

The diet is about 1,300 to 1,600 calories a day with the snack. When portion sizes are given as 3–4 ounces, men should choose the 4-ounce size, women the 3-ounce size. Men can have one extra snack

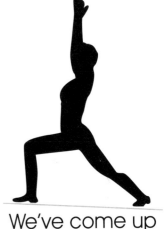

We've come up with some options that allow you to make substitutions that will work just as well.

a day from the snack list. Yes, it's unfair, but here's why: Men have more muscle than women, and are usually at a heavier body weight to begin with, so even with a weight loss program they will need more calories than women do. Remember what we said earlier about muscle burning more calories than fat? That extra muscle gives men the ability to consume more calories without going over their limit. Sorry, but it's just the way things are!

Do not be obsessive about the calorie counts. The quality of the calories is just as important as the number of calories, and the quality of the calories on this program is top-notch. This diet is designed to keep your blood sugar even, your energy levels constant, and to prevent your body from going into "fat storage" mode. Use it in conjunction with your scale. If you see your weight dropping at a consistent rate of about two pounds or so a week, it's working. If your weight is not moving, try making the portions slightly smaller, or cut out the snack. Remember that yoga is about consciousness, not perfection.

Here is the first of your six goals:

1. Eat mostly low-glycemic carbohydrates.

What are low-glycemic carbohydrates? Well, "glyco" means sugar, so in the simplest sense of the word, low glycemic means low sugar. But it's a little more complicated than that. Nutritionists used a tool called the glycemic index to measure exactly how fast blood sugar rises in response to a given food. Since blood sugar rises most in response to carbohydrates, carbohydrates are the foods that have been tested and rated on the glycemic index. The foods tested were compared to a dose of pure glucose, which gets a score of 100.

We don't want blood sugar to rise quickly because that will produce a surge of a hormone called *insulin*, a hormone which is responsible for storing fat rather than "burning" it. While the glycemic index is not a perfect measure—in fact, there are some foods with a high glycemic index that are quite good for you, and some with a low glycemic index that are not—it is still a decent guide to choosing foods that will not have a negative effect on your blood sugar and, subsequently, your fat-burning pathways. Nearly all of the carbohydrates chosen on the two-week plan are low glycemic, and those that are not are used sparingly and in small portions.

Recently, nutritionists have begun to use an even more sophisticated measure to determine how foods affect blood sugar and the subsequent hormonal cascade that can profoundly affect your weight. We call it the glycemic load. You see, some foods—like carrots, for example, or beets—have a high glycemic index and so have gotten a bad rap somewhat unfairly. Unfairly, because in point of fact you have to eat a lot of carrots, for example, to get make the blood sugar rise. The glycemic load takes into account the available carbohydrate in a typical portion size and then multiplies it by the glycemic index, resulting in a much more accurate picture of a food's blood-sugar-raising properties in the real world.

Here is a sample of the glycemic load of some common foods. Remember that in this list, low-glycemic foods are those having a glycemic load of 0 to 10, medium glycemic-load foods are those with a rating of 11 to 19, and high glycemic-load foods are those that are 20 or more. Whenever possible in choosing your foods, pick from lower glycemic-load foods. (If the glycemic load list isn't available but you happen to know the glycemic index, choose lower glycemic index foods rather than higher ones.)

LOW GLYCEMIC LOAD (10 OR FEWER)

- Strawberries: 1 (most berries are very low)
- Carrots: 3
- Watermelon: 4
- Cantaloupe: 4
- Pears: 4
- Beets: 5
- Oranges: 5
- Peaches: 5
- Red lentils: 5
- Apples: 6
- Kidney beans: 7
- All-Bran cereal: 8
- Chickpeas: 8
- Whole wheat flour bread: 9

MEDIUM GLYCEMIC LOAD (11 TO 19)

- White wheat flour bread: 11
- Apple juice: 11
- New potatoes: 12
- Bananas: 12

❙ Orange juice: 12
❙ Shredded wheat: 15
❙ Cheerios: 15
❙ Life cereal: 16
❙ Parboiled rice: 17
❙ Fettuccine: 18

HIGH GLYCEMIC LOAD (20 OR MORE)
❙ Spaghetti: 20
❙ Cornflakes: 21
❙ Linguine: 23
❙ White rice: 23
❙ Macaroni: 23
❙ Baked russet potatoes: 26

2. Eat a good balance of protein, the right kind of fats, and some carbohydrates at every meal.

We owe the popularization of this just-about-perfect eating pre-scription to Dr. Barry Sears, who championed it in the Zone books, and he was absolutely right. Fat has absolutely no effect on insulin, protein has some, carbohydrate has the most. You can get your blood sugar to behave like a soft, gentle lake rather than like the crashing waves of the Pacific Ocean by eating this way. Your goal is to prevent surges of quick energy (the famous "sugar rush") followed by lows of fatigue and even depression, inevitably followed by cravings for more sugar. And the best way to do this is to take your plate, imagine it in thirds, fill one-third with protein, and load the rest up with veg-etables (and the occasional fruit). Add a dollop of healthful fat—like avocado, nuts, olive oil, or butter—and you're in business! Keep the calories on the low side and you'll be on your way to creating a new you, not only in the way you look, but in the way you feel as well.

Remember, food is a drug—it has a profound effect on hormones and mood, and a balance of the kind described here is the surest way to get the best results.

3. Eat breakfast like a king, lunch like a prince, and dinner like a pauper.

This wonderful old truism is attributed to one of the early pio-neers of healthful eating, nutritionist Adele Davis, whose books are credited with bringing consciousness about food and health (and the term "health food") to public awareness. The theory behind it is simple: Your metabolism is most revved up and ready to go in the morning. This makes sense from an evolutionary point of view, because our ancestors literally awakened just as the sun rose and went to bed when it set. The workday was structured around daylight, because there was no electricity or artificial light to allow us to work or play at all hours as we do now. We were much more in touch with our circadian rhythms then than we are now. Now we are able to override these inherent biological cadences by all sorts of artificial means, from electric light to coffee, 24-hour diners, cities that never sleep, computers that are always on, and triple-shift workdays. Yoga is about getting back to what is essential and basic in you, and that includes the rhythms you are biologically programmed to respond to—the basic eternal rhythms of the earth, the moon, and the sun.

Since we are much more active and revved up in the morning, it makes far more sense to fuel our bodies in the best possible way at breakfast. Breakfast should be the biggest meal. (And it should never be skipped, by the way. Another of the four shared habits of the 3,000 successful people in the National Weight Control Registry study was that they never missed breakfast!) Lunch should be in the middle range as far as calories go. The 3 P.M. crash that so many of us experience on a regular basis is usually a result of eating simply too much food or too much carbohydrate, either of which is likely to send our blood sugar crashing and our energy into a nosedive. And, finally, dinner comes when we are winding down. Our metabolisms are settling in for the night and getting ready for the rest, recuperation, and renewal that our bodies need so desperately (and that we all too frequently do not provide). Dinner is not the time to stuff ourselves with food, even though that is what we conventionally do.

4. Eat slowly. You will feel fuller and be less hungry.

Grandma was right: Chew your food well, and chew it slowly. There's a physiological reason for this, and it actually will help you lose weight. Here's why: There's an appetite-regulating hormone called cholecystokinin—also known as CCK—which is released into the bloodstream from the upper small intestine. It stimulates gallbladder contraction and the secretion of pancreatic digestive

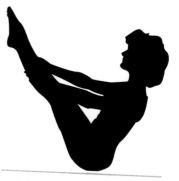

Yoga is about **getting back to what is** essential and basic in you.

enzymes. This hormone signals your brain that you have eaten enough. And it takes about 20 minutes to arrive at the brain. If you try eating a meal very slowly—as, for example, when you're engaged in really good, absorbing conversation—you will find that you're full on a lot less food. That's because you've given your body a chance to tell the brain "that's enough for now, we're finished down here!" Fast eaters never get the advantage of having that signal sent in time to stop eating. Their bodies are actually full long before the brain knows it. According to *The Hormone Revolution Weight-Loss Plan,* by Karlis Ullis, M.D., eating foods that boost insulin a lot, such as starchy carbohydrates (or those foods with a high glycemic load that we talked about earlier) do not promote the release of CCK and will cause you to become hungry again quickly. Dr. Ullis theorizes that this affects your appetite negatively in two ways: "1) It makes you consume more food and calories to feel full, and 2) the insulin stimulation causes your body to store the calories as fat." Bottom line: When eating, take your time!

5. Wait two hours after eating before going to bed.

Remember, large meals raise insulin levels, and if you go to bed with high levels of insulin circulating through your veins, you will not burn much fat during the night! Lighter meals should be the rule at dinner. And, if possible, try not eating after 7 or 8 P.M. If this just isn't practical, try to put as much awake time between your last meal and bedtime as you can, so that you are not regularly going to bed on a full stomach. You will see remarkable progress in your weight loss goals by following this simple suggestion.

6. Respect your body and its individuality.

Everyone is different. There's no reason you should feel that you're starving on this plan, but if you find yourself lightheaded, add a snack from the approved snack list. If you find yourself full on less food, simply cut out one of the snacks, or make the portions a bit smaller. You don't want to go too low in calories, though; this is completely counterproductive, because it sends a signal to the body that you're in a condition of deprivation. The body, in response, turns down its thermostat so that you can conserve energy for the starvation it is expecting. This is an ancient mechanism deeply programmed into our physiology as a survival strategy for times of famine. The body basically learns to go on a caloric budget and to make do with less. It learns to run on fewer calories, and it will conserve weight and hold on to fat. Then, when you begin eating "normally" again, it will grab on to every calorie it can and store it for when the next famine hits, causing a disheartening rebound. This is not a condition that you want to create. So don't go too low on calories thinking that if you can do with less your weight loss will move along that much faster. In the long run, such starvation tactics will work against you.

Your caloric needs may change somewhat from day to day depending on your activity level. If you do a particularly ambitious yoga practice—say, one of the 40-minute practices plus one of the 20-minute practices—and on the same day add some cardiovascular training, you may feel hungry on the plan and may need to augment it slightly. You can do this by taking somewhat larger portions or by adding a snack (or even two). Or you may feel just fine even with the added activity, and decide to stick with the plan exactly as is. Either is fine. A huge part of the success of this program comes from your ability to learn how to regulate your food intake depending on your actual energy needs, while at the same time learning to create just enough of a caloric deficit to create the weight loss you want. You will learn this over time by monitoring what you eat, weighing yourself, seeing how your clothes fit, and paying particular attention to things like your energy and your mood.

Follow this advice carefully: Honor your body's signals and learn to read them accurately. As Dr. Patty Ammon—a physician with fibromyalgia who lectures frequently on body-mind connections in the healing process—says, "The goal of the journey is to be present for the journey." Learn the difference between eating due to anxiety and eating due to real hunger. Learn to stop when full and to eat slowly enough to both appreciate the experience and to let your body tell you when it's had enough. Eventually you will be so in tune with who you are that what you want and what you need become the same thing.

Then you will have achieved something truly remarkable.

Chapter Eleven
The Two-Week Eating Plan

Success rests with the
courage, endurance, and,
above all, the will to become
the person you are, however
peculiar that may be. Then
you will be able to say,
"I have found my hero
and he is me."

—Dr. George Sheehan (runner and philosopher)

The two-week meal plan was created to get you started with "training wheels," like the kind you used when you first learned to ride a bicycle. We want you to think of it as an effortless way to begin thinking about food in a different way. It's effortless because everything is spelled out for you; follow it exactly and you will get excellent results, almost certainly drop a few pounds, and feel terrific. And it's a new way of thinking about food because, as you'll notice, many of the foods we've come to rely on heavily in the Western diet are either missing or severely reduced. There are only limited amounts of bread, small portions of rice, virtually no pasta, and limited cereals. (Remember: These foods were virtually absent in the human diet up until fairly recently in human history. The cavemen ate just fine without any of them!) The two-week plan is based on protein and vegetables and good fats, with the occasional portion of starch (usually from oatmeal or brown rice or whole grain bread).

If for some reason you need to substitute a different meal for one of the meals in the plan—for example, if you dine out one or two nights—that's fine. Try to stick to the spirit of the plan: Order lean protein (fish, turkey, chicken, or meat), a ton of vegetables, and add a dollop of good fat. (In the case of restaurant eating, olive oil or butter will do just fine.) If occasionally you need to have a starch, treat it as a condiment—have a small portion rather than making it the centerpiece of your meal (huge pasta plates, for example, are out). If you're going to have an occasional dessert, don't have it at the same meal as you're having a starch. And try to share it with another diner. The point is, you don't have to be slavish to any of the prescriptions found in this meal plan. It's a guide, included here for the purpose of getting you going on your own. However, you do have to maintain the spirit of consciousness about food that we have tried to stress throughout the book.

Note: Cooks, feel free to prepare and spice up the basics in any way you see fit. Most spices are rich sources of antioxidants and other beneficial compounds. Use them all you like.

Week One

As you begin week one of the eating plan, please remember that this is not a diet in the traditional sense of the word. First of all, you do not have to do it perfectly. Second, you want to look at these two weeks of menu choices as a set of guidelines and suggestions, not as a set of absolutes. (Don't forget, this is about "direction, not perfection"!)

Remember why you chose Molly Fox's Yoga Weight Loss Program in the first place? Something about its spirit connected with you. It's worth restating that spirit once again, so you can keep it firmly in mind as you embark on this new way of eating. This program is one of self-discovery, self-acceptance, and continual improvement in all areas of life (including, of course, the body). It is not about making judgments about your behavior, it is not about being "bad" or "good," and it does not include the word "cheating" in its vocabulary. We'd like you to approach this two-week set of suggestions with the spirit of inquiry and curiosity; think of it as one possible solution to the puzzle of "how do I combine lean quality protein, a huge amount of vegetables, good fats, and a limited amount of well-chosen starches and high-fiber/low-sugar fruits into meals for all situations?"

The purpose of this plan is not to give you a mindless prescription to follow, but to help you solve the problem of how to eat for the rest of your life in such a way that supports you in having a leaner, more youthful body and a more active, alive, and joyous being. It is meant as a teaching tool. If you approach it in this spirit, it will have more than served its purpose. Now have fun!

Day One

BREAKFAST

Dr. Baker's Wake-Up Protein Shake No. 1

This recipe is a favorite of mine and was originally used by the master educator, integrative physician, and author of *Detoxification and Healing,* Dr. Sid Baker.

YIELD: 1 SERVING

3 ounces skim or soy milk

3 ounces yogurt (full fat or low fat)

1 scoop whey or soy protein powder

1 tablespoon (or more) of ground flaxseed (flaxmeal)

¼ cup blueberries (or raspberries or blackberries)

4 ice cubes

In a blender, mix the milk and the yogurt. Add the scoop of protein powder, the flaxseed, and the blueberries. (For an even creamier feel, try using frozen berries. It will taste like an ice cream shake!) Add ice cubes and keep blending until thick and frosty. Serve right away.

LUNCH

Spicy Curry Grilled Chicken Breast Salad

This simple salad was designed as a foolproof throw-together by Chef Rick Starr, a Cordon Bleu chef. It's easy to prepare, incredibly simple, and extremely nutritious. It should give you a sense of what "eating clean" really means—combining nutritious, unprocessed foods consisting mainly of proteins and vegetables with some good fats included. Feel free to try your own variations; they are endless!

YIELD: 1 SERVING

4-ounce chicken breast (skinless, boneless)

Salt and pepper to taste

⅛ teaspoon curry powder

Pinch cayenne

Nonfat cooking spray or olive oil spray

5 ounces mixed green salad (use any combination of spinach leaves, arugula, lettuce, mushrooms, tomatoes/cherry tomatoes, red or green peppers)

2 tablespoons light vinaigrette salad dressing (storebought is fine; I suggest health food store brands like Amy's, which make terrific low-calorie dressings with virtually no additives, preservatives, or chemicals)

1. Preheat oven to 400 degrees. Season the breast with salt, pepper, curry powder, and cayenne. Coat a nonstick frying pan with nonfat cooking spray or olive oil spray. (You may use 1–2 tablespoons of extra-virgin olive oil, spread it around to coat the pan, and then blot up the rest.)

2. Heat the pan over medium heat. Pan-sear the seasoned chicken (for added color) until it is lightly browned on each side.

3. Finish in the oven until done, 25 minutes. Take out, let cool slightly, and cut into strips. Toss the green salad with vinaigrette and top with the strips of chicken.

Steak and Roasted Eggplant Salad

DINNER

Here's another way to combine lean protein with vegetables of your choice, this time featuring steak, eggplant, and spinach. Notice the small portion of beans—a healthy starch with lots of fiber, but fairly high calorically, hence the limited portion size. The combination should be satisfying and not leave you feeling heavy or sleepy.

YIELD: 1 SERVING

3–4 ounces lean sirloin

Salt and pepper to taste

1 tablespoon extra-virgin olive oil

Nonfat cooking spray or olive oil spray

1 cup

1 ounce romaine lettuce

1 ounce iceberg lettuce

1 ounce spinach leaves (organic, triple-washed is nice, but you can use regular as well)

2 tablespoons light salad dressing (you may use your choice of store-bought light dressings or you may make your own of oil and vinegar and spices. If you use a storebought dressing, choose one that has the least number of unpronounceable chemicals on the label as possible! This is why we recommend health food store brands.)

$3^2/_3$ cup cooked black beans (you can use canned as an alternative to fresh-cooked)

Steak and Roasted Eggplant Salad (continued)

1. Preheat oven to 400 degrees. Season steak with salt and pepper. Coat a nonstick frying pan with nonfat cooking spray or olive oil spray. (You may use 1–2 tablespoons of extra-virgin olive oil, spread it around to coat the pan, and then blot up the rest.) Heat the frying pan, medium high pan-sear the steak, and transfer to the oven to finish to desired doneness.

2. Brush the eggplant slices with olive oil and season to taste with salt and pepper. Grill or bake the eggplant in the oven until tender. Chop the lettuces and spinach, mix together, and top with the light salad dressing. Top the mixed greens with the black beans and seared steak.

Day Two

BREAKFAST

Homemade Breakfast Wrap

The unconventional breakfast choice that follows is a great example of thinking outside the box. The lettuce leaf makes a great "sandwich" that also travels well.

YIELD: 1 SERVING
Nonfat cooking spray or olive oil spray
½ bell pepper (red or green)
1 medium tomato
3–4 ounces chicken breast, cut into cubes or slices
1 tablespoon extra-virgin olive oil
1 large lettuce leaf

Coat a nonstick frying pan with the nonfat cooking spray or olive oil spray and heat. (You may use 1–2 tablespoons of extra-virgin olive oil, spread it around to coat the pan, and then blot up the rest.) Cut up the bell pepper into strips, and the tomato into slices. Quick stir-fry the cut-up chicken, and after a minute or so add the peppers and tomatoes until the chicken is done and the vegetables are bright colored and not too soft. Remove the mixture from the pan, drizzle with the tablespoon of olive oil, and wrap the mixture in a large lettuce leaf.

There is absolutely no reason why "dinner" foods can't be used for the first meal of the day. Foods like lean protein with vegetables have a wonderfully gentle effect on your blood sugar and will sustain you well for many hours, preventing that common 11 A.M. "crash." Strange as it sounds, Jonny frequently has salads for breakfast, often made with vegetables like spinach leaves, some berries, nuts, and olive oil. He feels energized and alert and ready to face the day!

Simple Tuna Salad

This basic staple can be made almost anywhere. You can carry a single-serving can of tuna with you to work, grab some salad from the salad bar (or bring it in a plastic container), throw the tuna over the greens, and complete your meal with an apple for dessert. If you can prepare the tuna salad at home, so much the better, as you can add spices, lemon juice, and, of course, extra-virgin olive oil as dressing.

YIELD: 1 SERVING

5 ounces mixed vegetables or premade salad (good choices include cherry tomatoes, mushrooms, spinach leaves, celery, and peppers)

3-ounce single-serving can tuna (you can even use the 6-ounce size and still wind up with a fairly low-calorie lunch!)

1 tablespoon extra-virgin olive oil as dressing

1 medium apple

Combine the vegetables and toss. Put the tuna on the vegetables, break into chunks, and toss salad again. Coat with the tablespoon of olive oil. Hint: you can eat the apple for dessert, but it also tastes delicious if you cut it up and add it to the salad.

Dill and Lime Halibut with Green Beans and Basmati Rice

The dill and lime give this fish dish a wonderful, fresh tropical taste.

YIELD: 1 SERVING

$^1/_3$ cup uncooked basmati rice (you may use brown rice instead if you like)

$^2/_3$ cup water

1 cup green beans

3–4 ounces halibut

Salt and pepper to taste

Fresh dill (to taste)

Nonfat cooking spray or olive oil spray

1 teaspoon

One lime wedge for garnish

1. Cook rice in boiling water according to directions until done. Steam or blanch the green beans to desired doneness. (They should be brightly colored and still slightly crisp.)

2. Season the halibut with salt and pepper and the fresh dill. Grill, broil, or pan-fry in a nonstick frying pan coated with nonfat cooking spray or olive oil spray. (You may use 1–2 tablespoons of extra-virgin olive oil, spread it around to coat the pan, and then blot up the rest.) Divide the pat of butter into two halves; put one half over the green beans and one half over the rice. As it melts, serve with the halibut. Garnish with the lime wedge, or squeeze the wedge over the fish before serving.

Day Three

Mixed Vegetables and Eggs

This is a favorite of Jonny's and is easy to throw together with any combination of vegetables you like. Use the ones listed as suggestions, but feel free to improvise. This is low-calorie, high-protein, high-fiber food at its best! Note: if you like, you can add a half grapefruit or a slice of gluten-free toast to accompany the egg dish.

YIELD: 2 SERVINGS

Nonfat cooking spray or olive oil spray

1 onion, sliced

1 green or red bell pepper, cut into slices

1 cup mushrooms, sliced

1 large tomato (or two small tomatoes), cut into small pieces

4 eggs, beaten (organic eggs from free-range chickens are best as they have the most omega-3 fatty acid content)

Salt and pepper to taste

▥ Coat a nonstick frying pan with nonfat cooking spray or olive oil spray. (You may use 1–2 tablespoons of extra-virgin olive oil, spread it around to coat the pan, and then blot up the rest.) Heat the pan and stir-fry the onion until it's transparent. Throw in the peppers, then the mushrooms, then the tomatoes. Stir-fry the mix until slightly softened. Pour the beaten eggs over the vegetables, mix with your spatula as it cooks, and continue to stir-fry until the eggs are done. Season with salt and pepper to taste, and serve.

Warning! Consuming raw or undercooked eggs is a potential health risk. Salmonella, a bacteria responsible for food poisoning, is one such result from raw or undercooked egg intake. Be aware of these potential health risks when preparing food.

Beef with Mixed Vegetables

LUNCH

Once again you have the option of choosing from an almost unlimited number of vegetables in any combination that you like. This is another easy way to combine lean protein with high-fiber, nutritious vegetables in a satisfying low-calorie dish. Broccoli looks and tastes really good in this dish. Jonny frequently uses a mix of broccoli and sweet red onions, which gives you a tremendous volume of food for very few calories. The sweetness of the onion mixes well with the slight tartness of the broccoli.

YIELD: 1 SERVING

3–4 ounces lean beef or chopped steak

Salt and pepper to taste

6 ounces mixed vegetables, cut for steaming

1 teaspoon butter

Beef with Mixed Vegetables (continued)

▓ Season the beef with salt and pepper, then broil until done. (Alternately, you can pan-fry in a nonstick frying pan coated with nonfat cooking spray or olive oil spray.) Steam the mixed vegetables until done (look for brightness of color), add salt and pepper to taste, melt the pat of butter over the vegetables, and serve with the meat.

DINNER

Cracked White Pepper Pork Tenderloin with Cauliflower and Sweet Potato Fries

Sweet potatoes, though a starchy carbohydrate, are nonetheless one of the most nutritious foods on the planet. They are loaded with antioxidants (a class of vitamins and minerals that help prevent or counteract damage at the cellular level and have been widely studied for a variety of beneficial effects on human health), plus they taste great. Sweet potatoes are always preferable to regular old white potatoes! If you don't like cauliflower, you can substitute any cruciferous vegetable (like broccoli or Brussels sprouts) or you can simply make a mixed green salad and toss it with a tablespoon of light vinaigrette dressing.

YIELD: 1 SERVING
1 small sweet potato (or yam)
Salt and pepper to taste
Extra-virgin olive oil
3–4 ounces pork tenderloin
1 teaspoon cracked or coarsely ground white pepper
Nonfat cooking spray or olive oil spray
4 ounces cauliflower (see above for substitutions)
Pinch of fresh herbs, minced
1 teaspoon butter

1. Heat oven to 400 degrees. Peel potato and slice into ¼"-thick pieces. Cut into "fries," brush with olive oil, season with the salt and pepper, and bake until done. (You should be able to put a fork through the "fries.")

2. Season the tenderloin with salt, and press ½ teaspoon cracked pepper on one side. Coat a sauté pan with nonfat cooking spray or olive oil spray, heat medium to high and sear the pepper side of the

steak. Remove from the pan, press the remaining cracked pepper on the other side, and sear. Finish in oven until desired doneness.

Steam or blanch the cauliflower until tender, and toss with the pat of butter, fresh herbs, and salt and pepper. Serve together.

Jonny's Favorite Morning Shake

Protein shakes can be a veritable laboratory for your creative juices. Here's one with a couple of unconventional "add-ons" that give it both flavor and texture.

YIELD: 1 SERVING

6–8 ounces water

1 scoop soy or whey protein powder

2 tablespoons old-fashioned oatmeal

1 tablespoon almond (or peanut) butter

1 tablespoon ground flaxseed (flaxmeal)

4 ice cubes

||| Place all ingredients in a blender. Blend until thick and frothy. Serve immediately.

Sardine Salad for One

Sardines are one of the unsung heroes of the health food world. Cheap, easy, portable, and readily available, they are literally packed with good stuff like healthful fats (omega-3 fatty acids) and high-quality protein.

YIELD: 1 SERVING

Large green mixed salad (any combination of mixed lettuces, peppers, mushrooms, tomatoes, broccoli, cauliflower, carrots, or other available vegetables of your choosing)

1 can sardines (packed in water, olive oil, or tomato sauce)

Salt and pepper to taste

1 tablespoon extra-virgin olive oil (you can omit this if you use sardines packed in olive oil)

||| Toss the vegetables together, add the sardines, season to taste, mix lightly, and top with the olive oil for dressing. Enjoy!

DINNER

Herbed Chicken Breast

This is another way to combine lean protein with green vegetables and a small portion of starch. This easy and nutritious meal is low in calories and high in nutrients.

YIELD: 1 SERVING

4–5 ounces boneless, skinless chicken breast
2 tablespoons extra-virgin olive oil
1 ounce blanched almonds (you can use slivered or raw almonds as well)
$1/3$ cup uncooked basmati rice (or brown rice)
1 cup broccoli florets
Salt and pepper to taste
Fresh minced herbs (your choice)

1. Preheat oven to 400 degrees. Rub the chicken with 1 tablespoon of the olive oil, add half the almonds, and season to taste. Bake until juice runs clear when pricked with a fork, about 20 minutes.

2. Cook the rice in water according to package directions, until done. Blanch or steam the broccoli; when done, toss with remaining tablespoon of olive oil and the other half of the almonds. Season with salt, pepper, and minced herbs. Serve the chicken with broccoli and rice on the side.

Day Five

BREAKFAST

Basic Traditional Breakfast with a Healthful Twist

There are a lot of ways to combine bread, fruit, protein, and good fats. This is one of them. It is much better for you than the "traditional" combination of buttered bread, cereal, and orange juice, but not so very different that if you're used to the "usual" you can't adapt to this much better option.

1 SERVING

$1/2$ grapefruit
One slice gluten-free toast
1 tablespoon almond butter
3 ounces yogurt

IIII Serve the grapefruit as a first course. Spread the almond butter over the gluten-free toast and serve accompanied by the yogurt. Jonny likes the yogurt spread over the almond-buttered bread and eaten together. It's delicious either way.

Deviled Ham–Tuna Salad Combination

LUNCH

This recipe takes about 5 minutes to prepare once you've got the hard-boiled eggs. You can serve one mound as an appetizer, or make a lunch out of a two-mound serving.

YIELD: 2 SERVINGS OF TWO MOUNDS EACH

4 ounces finely chopped cooked lean ham

$6\frac{1}{2}$-ounce can drained water-packed tuna, drained, broken into small flakes

2 hard-boiled eggs, chopped

1 tablespoon dill pickle relish

1 teaspoon onion flakes

2 teaspoons lemon juice

$\frac{1}{2}$ teaspoon paprika

Allspice to taste

Lemon wedges

IIII Combine all ingredients except the last two with a fork. Arrange in four mounds, dusting tops lightly with a little allspice, and add a lemon wedge alongside each.

Lemon Pepper Salmon

DINNER

You can't beat salmon as a source of protein and good fats rolled into one. And kale has the highest antioxidant rating of any vegetable.

YIELD: 1 SERVING

1 small sweet potato

3–4 ounces salmon (boneless fillet or steaks)

Salt and cracked black pepper to taste

1 teaspoon butter

1 teaspoon lemon juice

$\frac{1}{2}$ tablespoon extra-virgin olive oil

1 clove garlic, peeled, then chopped or minced

6 ounces spinach or kale (rinse well; dry)

Lemon Pepper Salmon (continued)

1. Bake the sweet potato at 375 degrees until tender.

2. Season the salmon with the salt and pepper and top with the butter. Bake the salmon at 400 degrees until desired doneness is reached; squeeze a little lemon juice over the fish before serving.

3. Meanwhile, in a sauté pan, heat the olive oil and sauté the garlic until fragrant. Add the kale (or spinach); stir until just wilted. Serve the kale with the potato and the salmon.

Salmon is a great weight-loss food and should occupy a regular place in this program. If you have a choice, wild salmon is best, though it's harder to find than the more common farm-raised. Remember, while you're on the two-week eating plan (as opposed to when you're simply trying to maintain your desired weight), portions should be kept as close to the 3- or 4-ounce size as possible when you dine out. Most restaurant portions are much larger. Take the rest of the salmon home! It's great cold on a green salad.

Day Six

BREAKFAST **Variation on the American Cowboy Breakfast**

There is simply no better breakfast food than eggs, and no, they will not have any significant effect on your blood cholesterol! Jonny recommends that you eat the whole egg, not just the white. There are an endless number of ways to prepare eggs. Here's a sample of how to put together your favorite style of eggs with a fruit and a starch in a winning combination, devoid of the usual "potatoes, bacon, white bread, and juice" that frequently accompany this perfect food (and in the process turn it into a nutritional nightmare).

YIELD: 1 SERVING

2 eggs, cooked, any style (scrambled, poached, boiled)

1 slice gluten-free toast

$\frac{1}{3}$ cup berries (blueberries, raspberries, blackberries, or strawberries)

|||| Cook the eggs in your favorite style and serve with the gluten-free toast and berries accompaniment. If you scramble the eggs, feel free to throw in some vegetables like onions, mushrooms, or peppers, or use vegetables to make an omelet.

Warning! Consuming raw or undercooked eggs is a potential health risk. Salmonella, a bacteria responsible for food poisoning, is one such result from raw or undercooked egg intake. Be aware of these potential health risks when preparing food.

Homemade Easy Tuna for One

LUNCH

The secret ingredient in this tuna salad is the apple. While the celery provides crunchiness, the apple provides juiciness and sweetness that is unexpected in a tuna salad and creates a delightful taste sensation.

YIELD: 1 SERVING

2 stalks celery

1 red pepper

1 small apple

1 can tuna, packed in water, drained (you can use the 3-ounce single-serving size or, if you're hungry, a whole 6-ounce can)

1 tablespoon extra-virgin olive oil (you may substitute homemade mayo)

Lemon juice to taste

Red pepper to taste

Large leaf of lettuce

Homemade Easy Tuna for One (continued)

⁍ Chop the celery, pepper, and apple. Mix together and measure out 1 to 2 cups of the mixture. (Reserve the remainder for another day or another salad.) Mix the tuna in with the vegetables and top with the tablespoon of olive oil (or homemade mayo), lemon juice, and pepper. Serve on a large leaf of lettuce.

DINNER

Ginger Chicken and Grapes

This recipe was a favorite of the ladies on Jonny's iVillage "Shape Up" community challenge, who passed it around the Internet as part of an impromptu "cookbook" of "Shape-Up" friendly recipes. It fits in perfectly with our philosophy of fresh, minimally processed food containing protein, lots of vegetables, good fats, and small amounts of starches and fruits.

YIELD: 1 SERVING
Extra-virgin olive oil for stir-frying
4 ounces boneless, skinless chicken, cut into strips
2 cups mixed broccoli, snow peas, onions
Fresh ginger, grated to taste
1 cup seedless red grapes

⁍ Coat a nonstick frying pan with olive oil. Heat the pan and sauté all the ingredients except the grapes, turning and mixing with a spatula frequently until chicken is browned and tender and the vegetables are done. Serve on a plate with the cup of seedless grapes.

Day Seven

BREAKFAST

The Bodybuilder's Special

This combination—in some form or another—has been a standard favorite of bodybuilders for years. The reason? High-quality protein (the egg), and a good carbohydrate with a lot of fiber (the oatmeal). Though bodybuilders usually eat significantly greater portion sizes than the ones found here, you can get the same competitive edge out of this breakfast as they do, albeit in a lower calorie (smaller portion) version.

The Bodybuilder's Special (continued)

TIP: Instead of having to choose between the butter and the half and half, you can get the best of both worlds by mixing ½ teaspoon butter and half as a topping for your oatmeal.

Remember not to use the single-serving "packets" of oatmeal or the "1 minute instant" kind. Neither is nearly as nutritious as the old-fashioned "slow cooking" kind, which really doesn't take much longer to make than the packets!

YIELD: 1 SERVING
1 teaspoon
1 cup cooked oatmeal
Cinnamon to taste
Salt and pepper to taste
1 hard-boiled egg

Put the butter (or half and half) on the oatmeal, mix together, season with cinnamon, salt, and pepper, and serve alongside the egg. Of course, you can season the egg with the salt and pepper as well.

Grilled Chicken Salad

LUNCH

There are endless ways to put together lean meat, poultry, or fish with vegetables. Feel free to improvise, using this recipe as a guide.

YIELD: 1 SERVING
3–4 ounces cooked chicken breast, sliced
1 cup green or romaine lettuce
½ cup broccoli florets
1 cup red pepper strips
1 medium tomato or 1 cup cherry tomatoes
1 tablespoon extra-virgin olive oil
Lemon juice to taste
Vinegar to taste
Salt and freshly ground black pepper to taste

Grilled Chicken Salad (continued)

IIII In a large salad bowl combine the chicken, lettuce, broccoli, pepper, and tomatoes. Top with olive oil, lemon juice, vinegar, and salt and pepper and toss again before serving.

DINNER

Citrus Flavored Juicy Halibut Steak

This is a light fish loaded with nutrients. Serve this with your choice of any steamed vegetable, or accompany it with a nice mixed green salad.

YIELD: 4 SERVINGS

2 halibut steaks (total about 2 pounds) approximately $1\frac{1}{4}$ to $1\frac{1}{2}$ inches thick

$\frac{1}{2}$ teaspoon salt

$\frac{1}{4}$ teaspoon mixed herbs (your choice)

$\frac{1}{2}$ cup unsweetened grapefruit juice

$\frac{1}{2}$ teaspoon paprika

4 thin slices lemon

1. Preheat broiler. Wipe halibut steaks with wet paper towels and place on foil in broiler pan. Mix together salt, herbs, and grapefruit juice, and brush this mixture over the fish. Sprinkle with paprika and broil about 3 inches from the heat until the fish is just browned (about 6 minutes).

2. Turn fish, brush again with juice, and sprinkle with paprika. Broil 5 minutes, basting with the juice once or twice. Place 2 lemon slices over the top of each steak, return to the broiler, and broil for 2 minutes longer. Fish should flake easily with a fork, but do not overcook. Cut steaks in half to serve.

Week Two

By now you should be getting the hang of preparing your food according to the principles of the Yoga Weight Loss Program. You may have noticed that all the recipes and suggestions for the week-one menu were relatively simple, straightforward, and easy to prepare. The key ingredients to every meal: protein, vegetables (or the occasional fruit), and good-quality fats like olive oil or butter (or avocado, nuts, flaxseed oil, and the like).

By the end of the second week you will be well on your way to losing weight and, more important, learning a new way of seeing food as both a fuel for your body and also as a source of joy and pleasure. When food is fairly "clean" like the recipes in the two-week plan (i.e., free of sauces, sugars, and other "taste distracters") you will also develop an appreciation of what foods can really taste like when they are fresh, prepared with care and consciousness, not over-cooked, and not overseasoned.

Day Eight

Banana Egg Cream

BREAKFAST

This high-protein drink is one of Jonny's absolute favorites, and is especially good when you don't have a lot of time. Don't gulp it down, though; it's just too good not to enjoy slowly.

YIELD: 1 SERVING
4 ounces banana
5 large egg whites
1 egg
6 ounces 2% milk
(optional) 3 or 4 ice cubes

Put all ingredients into a blender and blend until thick and frothy.

TIP: This tastes even better if the banana has been frozen overnight. If you do freeze it, peel it first and cut it into 4-ounce pieces!

LUNCH   **Turkey and Avocado**

Many people avoid avocado because they think it's "fattening." In fact, avocado contains one of the best kinds of fat on the planet, and it's a terrific idea to have small amounts of it in your diet on a regular basis. The trick is not to overindulge. A little piece of interesting trivia should you ever find yourself on the *Jeopardy* TV game show: avocados are fruits, not vegetables.

YIELD: 1 SERVING

3–4 ounces sliced turkey breast (fresh turkey is best, but good deli turkey will definitely do)
¼ small avocado, thinly sliced
3 slices tomato
Dijon mustard to taste
2 leaves romaine lettuce
1 sliced carrot
½ red pepper, chopped
1 kiwi, sliced
10 red raspberries

||| On a plate or in a salad bowl combine the turkey, the avocado, and the tomato. Season with Dijon mustard to taste. Arrange on the two leaves of romaine lettuce.

In a separate bowl combine the sliced carrot and the ½ cup chopped red pepper and toss together. Serve the carrot/pepper mixture as an accompaniment to the turkey salad. For dessert, serve the sliced kiwi decorated with the raspberries.

DINNER   **Tofu Pita Pizza**

Who says you can't ever have your favorite foods on a weight loss program? The trick is to make carefully chosen healthful substitutions, watch the portion size, and don't indulge too frequently.

This recipe will satisfy your cravings for pizza. Some of Jonny's clients say that they now like it better than the "real" thing!

Tofu Pita Pizza (continued)

YIELD: 1 SERVING

3 ounces crumbled firm tofu

$\frac{1}{2}$ teaspoon minced garlic

$\frac{1}{2}$ cup tomato sauce

$\frac{1}{2}$ cup chopped broccoli (fresh or frozen)

$\frac{1}{4}$ cup chopped fresh tomato

1 whole wheat or whole grain pita (6 inches, unopened)

One medium apple

Heat oven to 400 degrees. Mix the tofu with the garlic. Layer tomato sauce, chopped broccoli, chopped fresh tomato, and tofu mixture on pita, and heat through in oven. For dessert, serve the apple.

Day Nine

BREAKFAST

All-American with a Healthy Twist

Jonny uses this one a lot with his private nutrition clients, particularly those who are used to "conventional" breakfasts of cereal and milk. The problem with most of those conventional "low-fat" breakfasts is that they are very high in sugar, have almost no protein, and don't keep you satisfied or energized for long. Here's a variation that corrects those deficits while adding a few special touches in the bargain.

YIELD: 1 SERVING

$\frac{1}{2}$ grapefruit

2 ounces whole grain high-fiber cereal
    (such as All-Bran or Fiber One)

6 raw almonds

3–4 ounces soy or skim milk

Unsweetened shredded coconut

1 hard- or soft-boiled egg

Salt and pepper to taste

Serve the grapefruit first. Mix the cereal with the almonds. Pour the milk on top of the cereal mixture and sprinkle with the coconut. Season the egg with salt and pepper to taste. Serve the cereal with the egg on the side.

LUNCH

Tuna Sandwich with Berry Dessert

In general, this program is not big on bread for several reasons. One, it is very high in carbs; two, it is high glycemic (see Chapter 10 for a full explanation of the glycemic load); three, bread is very easy to overeat; and four, many people are sensitive to wheat. This is one of only four sandwiches you'll see in the two-week eating plan. All things considered, it's a good choice.

YIELD: 1 SERVING
4 ounces albacore tuna, packed in water, drained
2 teaspoons Dijon mustard
2 tablespoons chopped celery
2 tablespoons chopped onion
1 teaspoon fresh chopped dill (or ¼ teaspoon dried)
6-inch whole wheat or whole grain pita
2 pieces of dark leaf lettuce
2 slices tomato
1 cup of fresh berries (blackberries, blueberries, raspberries, or strawberries)

Combine the tuna with the Dijon mustard, the chopped celery, the chopped onion, and the dill. Stuff the combination into the pita and add the 2 pieces of dark leaf lettuce and 2 slices of tomato. Serve. Enjoy the fresh berries for dessert.

DINNER

Chicken Stir-Fry with Apple

YIELD: 1 SERVING
Nonfat cooking spray or olive oil spray
1 tablespoon minced garlic
1 cup small broccoli florets
½ red pepper, sliced
1–2 tablespoons water
3–4 ounces cubed chicken breast (uncooked)
1 medium apple

Coat a nonstick skillet with nonfat cooking spray or olive oil spray. (You may use 1–2 tablespoons of extra-virgin olive oil, spread it around to coat the pan, and then blot up the rest.) Sauté the garlic for 30 seconds over medium-high heat. Add the broccoli florets, red bell pepper, and 1–2 tablespoons water; stir-fry for 2 to 3 minutes. Add the chicken; stir and cook for another 3 to 5 minutes or until the chicken turns golden. Serve. Finish with the apple for dessert.

Day Ten

BREAKFAST

Jonny's Special High Protein Oatmeal

Here's a great way to beef up regular oatmeal with more protein for a more complete one-dish breakfast.

YIELD: 1 SERVING

2 ounces old-fashioned oatmeal

Water as needed

¾ cup nonfat or soy milk

1 scoop whey or soy protein powder

Cinnamon to taste

1 tablespoon slivered almonds

||| Put the oatmeal in a microwavable bowl, add enough water to cover it plus just a little more, and microwave on medium heat for 4 minutes. Remove from microwave and stir, adding a little more water if necessary if you like it a little thinner. Add the scoop of protein powder and the milk and mix well. If necessary, add a little more water. Season liberally with cinnamon and sprinkle on the slivered almonds.

TIP: Vanilla protein powder mixes really well and creates an interesting taste sensation.

Veggie Burger with Salad

LUNCH

Veggie burgers are now widely available in restaurants and can be purchased in patty form in the frozen foods sections of many supermarkets, especially those with health food sections. While this program is hardly against the use of lean meats (or poultry or eggs for that matter), a vegetarian version of the standard hamburger is a nice change of pace.

YIELD: 1 SERVING

1 cup mixed greens (premade salad, or choose from spinach leaves, arugula, lettuce, dark lettuces, romaine lettuce, cherry tomatoes, asparagus, broccoli florets, mushrooms, julienne sliced carrots)

Veggie Burger with Salad (continued)

2½ tablespoons chickpeas (or other available bean)
1 tablespoon balsamic vinegar
One veggie burger (from frozen food department)
One multigrain bun
Lettuce leaves (to cover burger)
Large fresh tomato, cut into thin slices

1. Toss the salad with the chickpeas and the balsamic vinegar.

2. Grill the veggie burger (or pan-fry in a nonstick frying pan with nonfat cooking spray) until desired state of doneness. (Hint: Don't overcook. Veggie burgers usually don't require as much time in the pan as their real meat counterparts.) Serve the burger on the multigrain bun with lettuce and the tomato slices, accompanied by the salad.

TIP: You can leave out the bun if you like and eat this as a veggie burger platter, thus cutting down on your intake of bread.

DINNER

Poached Salmon Steaks with Dill Sauce

Combine this delicious salmon dish with a 6-ounce serving of the vegetable of your choice for a perfect low-calorie, high-protein meal. The portion size of the salmon is a little bigger than we've been using so far, but the absence of a starch makes up for the additional calories. Besides, it's hard to find salmon steaks of less than 5 to 6 ounces.

YIELD: 4 SERVINGS
1 cup water
1 cup chicken bouillon
½ teaspoon dill seed
½ teaspoon chopped fresh dill
¼ teaspoon seasoned salt
1 bay leaf
Lemon slices
4 salmon steaks, about 6 ounces each

1. Combine all ingredients except salmon steaks in a large saucepan, and bring to a boil. Add salmon and bring to boil again, then reduce heat and simmer about 4 minutes, or until salmon flakes easily.

2. Serve salmon steaks on warm platter, sprinkling a little more chopped fresh dill over them. May be served with the following:

Dill Sauce

$^1/_2$ cup regular cottage cheese
3 tablespoons canned onion broth
$1^1/_2$ teaspoons snipped fresh dill
Salt and pepper to taste

|||| Combine all ingredients in a blender and process at low speed until creamy and smooth.

TIP: This sauce is great with salmon, but it also tastes terrific with other fish. If you're figuring calories, each tablespoon is about 15.

Day Eleven

Homemade Muesli and Hard-Boiled Egg

BREAKFAST

Many of Jonny's private nutrition clients are surprised to learn that they can actually eat oatmeal raw, but raw oats are the main ingredient of the traditional Swiss cereal known as muesli, which you can now buy by the box in almost any grocery store. As a snack, Jonny frequently sprinkles raw oats on a variety of fruit and nut combinations and eats it either dry or with a little bit of milk.

YIELD: 1 SERVING
2 ounces slow-cooking oats
1 ounce raisins (or dates)
1 ounce almonds (raw is best)
3 ounces soy milk
1 hard-boiled egg
Unsweetened shredded coconut mix to taste

|||| Soak the oats, raisins, and almonds in the soy milk until soft (about 10 minutes). Sprinkle with the unsweetened coconut. Serve with the hard-boiled egg on the side.

Chicken Vegetable Soup with Melon Dessert

Jonny actually came up with this as a solution to his elderly parents' dilemma of what to eat for dinner when they weren't very hungry. Older folks often don't feel as hungry or thirsty and feel full on very little food, putting them in danger of being seriously undernourished at a time when they need all the nutritional bang for the buck they can possibly get. While usually we don't love the idea of canned soups (we hope you will prefer to make your own when time permits), this is a great way to turn a can of soup into a nutritious meal with minimum effort.

> YIELD: 1 SERVING
> ¾ cup cooked mixed frozen vegetables
> 1 cup chicken vegetable soup (such as Campbell's
>   Healthy Request)
> 2 ounces of roasted chicken breast
> Salt and pepper to taste
> 1 cup fresh honeydew melon

1. Microwave the vegetables (in just enough water to make a little bed for the vegetables) in bowl covered until they are thawed and just slightly done.

2. Heat the soup. Add the vegetables and the chicken breast. Stir, heat to desired temperature, season to taste, and serve. Have the honeydew melon for dessert.

Roasted Pork Chop with Green Beans and Potatoes

Pork is a great substitute for chicken. Just make sure it's trimmed of fat and cooked until brown, about 25 to 30 minutes. You can, of course, substitute any green vegetable for the green beans.

> YIELD: 1 SERVING
> 1 4-ounce pork chop, trimmed of fat
> Nonfat cooking spray or olive oil spray
> Salt and pepper to taste
> 3 ounces cubed potatoes
> 1 pat (1 tablespoon) butter
> Chopped fresh parsley to taste
> 1 to 1½ cup green beans

Roasted Pork Chop with Green Beans and Potatoes (continued)

1. Preheat oven to 350 degrees. Coat a nonstick skillet with nonfat cooking spray or olive oil spray. (You may use 1–2 tablespoons of extra-virgin olive oil, spread it around to coat the pan, and then blot up the rest.)

2. Heat the skillet over medium-high heat. Season pork chop with salt and pepper, and pan-sear in the hot skillet. Bake in the oven covered for 30 minutes.

3. Meanwhile, boil the cubed potatoes until tender. Drain; add butter, salt, pepper, and parsley, and mix thoroughly.

4. Steam or blanch the green beans and season with salt and pepper. Serve meat, potatoes, and vegetables together.

Day Twelve

BREAKFAST

Simple Shaker Breakfast

Here is another way to combine basic ingredients with virtually no preparation time. The yogurt provides the protein, the almond butter provides the good fat, and the apple and the bread (especially if you choose carefully from health food store brands like Ezekiel) provide the fiber and good carbs.

YIELD: 1 SERVING
1 tablespoon natural peanut butter (or almond butter)
1 slice 7-grain bread (even better: sprouted grain or Ezekiel bread)
8 ounces vanilla nonfat yogurt
1 medium apple

‖ Spread the nut butter on the bread and serve with the yogurt and apple on the side.

Egg Mock-Sandwich with Fruit Smoothie

LUNCH

Using one slice of bread cuts down on the carbs and calories and results in a lunch with plenty of high-quality protein as well as low-sugar fruit. Feel free to add a mixed green salad with a tablespoon of extra-virgin olive oil as an accompaniment.

Egg Mock-Sandwich with Fruit Smoothie (continued)

YIELD: 1 SERVING

Nonfat cooking spray or olive oil spray

2 eggs

Salt and pepper to taste

1 slice Ezekiel or sprouted grain bread

1 tomato, sliced

1 cup frozen blueberries

½ cup skim milk or low-fat vanilla soy milk

1. Scramble the eggs in a nonstick fry pan coated with nonfat cooking spray or olive oil spray. Season to taste with salt and pepper.

2. Toast the bread. Serve the eggs on the toast, and top with tomato slices. Blend the milk and the berries in a blender and serve as dessert.

DINNER

Baked Greek Island Chicken

Simple recipe, but bursting with flavors that take you to the Greek Islands right in your own kitchen! Developed by Chef Patti Hulsey of Santa Monica, California, especially for this program!

YIELD: 1 SERVING

4-ounce chicken breast, skinless

1 teaspoon Greek seasoning

½ cup water

2 Roma tomatoes, diced

1 yellow onion, sliced

¼ medium green pepper, sliced

½ zucchini, sliced thin

2 tablespoons sliced black Greek olives

3 cloves fresh garlic, coarsely chopped

1 teaspoon oregano

Salt and pepper to taste

1. Preheat oven to 350 degrees. Season chicken breast on all sides with Greek seasoning. Place in shallow baking dish with ¼ cup of water. Bake uncovered for 10 minutes. Remove from oven; set aside.

2. Toss Roma tomatoes, onion, peppers, and zucchini together, adding olives, garlic, and oregano. Arrange vegetables around chicken

Baked Greek Island Chicken (continued)

breast in the baking dish. Add ¼ cup of water. Place back in oven and bake for another 15 minutes. Season to taste with salt and pepper.

Day Thirteen

"Protein Been Berry Berry Good to Me" Shake

BREAKFAST

Protein shakes are a constant in the nutritional arsenal of the on-the-go person. With a little creative thinking and a blender at work, you can use them as an afternoon pick-me-up as well as a mini-meal or a full-scale breakfast substitute. The ice cubes add bulk, frothiness, and texture.

YIELD: 1 SERVING

4 ounces blueberries (or strawberries)
1 whole egg
2 large egg whites
4 ounces 2% milk
1 scoop protein powder (whey or soy)
4 ice cubes (optional)

Combine all ingredients in a blender. Add ice cubes if desired. Blend until thick and frothy.

Tuna Sandwich with Sweet Relish

LUNCH

Tuna is a great timesaver and can be prepared so many different ways. This version travels really well in a lunch bag or a plastic container.

YIELD: 1 SERVING

3–4 ounces white albacore tuna, packed in water, drained
1 teaspoon Dijon mustard
1 teaspoon sweet relish
Freshly squeezed juice from 1 lemon wedge
1 whole wheat or whole grain pita
2 pieces dark leaf lettuce
2 slices tomato

Mix the tuna with the Dijon mustard, the relish, and the lemon juice. Combine and stuff into pita. Add the lettuce and the tomato.

Beef Tenderloin with Asparagus and Baked Potato

The beauty of tenderloin is that you don't have to do anything to it. With this dish, feel free to skip the potatoes and substitute a second vegetable such as grilled red peppers (or load up on extra asparagus).

YIELD: 1 SERVING

3–4 ounces beef tenderloin
Salt and pepper to taste
Nonfat cooking oil spray
$1/2$ tablespoon extra-virgin olive oil
4 ounces fresh asparagus
1 teaspoon
¾ cup unsweetened applesauce

1. Bake the potato at 400 degrees until tender.

2. Season the tenderloin with salt and pepper. Coat a sauté pan with nonfat cooking spray, add the olive oil, and over medium-high heat, sear the seasoned meat. Sear on both sides for color only, and finish in the oven to desired doneness.

3. Grill, blanch, or pan-fry the asparagus in a nonstick fry pan coated with nonfat cooking spray. Season the asparagus with salt, pepper, and $1/2$ of the butter. Use the remaining butter on the potato. Serve together with applesauce on the side.

Day Fourteen

BREAKFAST

Jason's Perfect Egg and Avocado Mix

By now you should be getting the idea that eggs can be a staple on this program, and that there are endless ways to prepare them and combine them with other foods. This is a simple way to get protein and fiber in a very basic breakfast that takes hardly any time to prepare.

YIELD: 1 SERVING

2 hard-boiled eggs
Approximately $1/4$ of a small avocado
One medium tomato, diced
Salt and pepper to taste
One cup fresh spinach leaves (washed)

Jason's Perfect Egg and Avocado Mix (continued)

1. Put the eggs in a pot of water and bring to a rolling boil. Let the boil continue for 30 seconds. Then turn off the flame and set the timer to 12 minutes. The eggs will be perfectly done.

2. Peel and chop the eggs. Peel the avocado, and chop into small pieces. Mix the egg, avocado, and diced tomato together, season to taste, and serve over the bed of spinach leaves.

Cup of Soup with Yogurt Dessert

Sometimes you have to improvise with what you have around, especially when time is a factor. Choices like this liberate you from having to be a prisoner to the food court or fast-food restaurant choices. It takes a minute to put together and you can take it with you!

YIELD: 1 SERVING

1 cup minestrone soup (single serving "on-the-go" cup such as Fantastic Foods or Health Valley)
1 scoop whey or soy protein powder
1 cup plain nonfat yogurt
$\frac{1}{2}$ cup fresh or frozen berries

▥ Prepare soup according to the package directions. Mix in the scoop of protein powder and stir until dissolved. Mix the yogurt with the berries for dessert.

Take-Out Shrimp and Vegetables

Molly Fox's Yoga Weight Loss Program is about being able to make conscious choices no matter what the circumstances. Here's a way, for example, to make a healthy dinner when the family goes out for Chinese food or orders take-out food. A great weight loss program trick is to order sauce on the side and simply dip your fork into it as you eat, rather than pouring the whole amount over the food.

YIELD: 1 SERVING

$\frac{1}{2}$ cup hot and sour soup
4 ounces steamed shrimp (approximately 6–8 medium- to large-sized)
$1\frac{1}{2}$ cups steamed snow peas (or other vegetable such as broccoli)
$\frac{1}{2}$ cup brown rice
2 tablespoons sweet and sour orange sauce (optional)

Take-Out Shrimp and Vegetables (continued)

||| Start your meal with the hot and sour soup. Follow with the shrimp and the vegetable, mixed and served over the rice. Optional: Top with 2 tablespoons sweet and sour sauce.

Snacks

The accepted conventional wisdom of most weight loss programs is that it is best to eat small meals frequently, which usually comes out to be three meals and two snacks. This allows you to eat every three to four hours and prevents your blood sugar from going too low and setting you up for crashes and cravings, which can sabotage virtually any weight loss program. At the same time, keeping meals small and balanced (i.e., not overly high in carbohydrates, with each meal containing some protein and good fat) helps to keep insulin levels from skyrocketing.

So snacks are an important part of your diet, and you should make full use of them. Unlike most snacks, which are junk foods— conveniently packaged but loaded with calories and sugar and virtually devoid of nutritional goodies—these snacks are very much in keeping with Molly Fox's Yoga Weight Loss Program. Have up to two a day. You can eat them whenever you like, but a good idea is to space them between your meals so that you never go more than four hours without eating something.

It's not a disaster if you find yourself not eating one (or even, occasionally, both) of the snacks. You may find that because the meals you are preparing are so nutritious, you are actually not as hungry between meals as you once were. The snacks are there to give you options and to be used as needed.

A Note about Oil

In the recipe section of the book, you may have noticed an almost exclusive reliance on extra-virgin olive oil. This is because it is one of the best oils for cooking, and contains heart-healthy monounsaturated fats. Extra-virgin simply means that it is cold-pressed. This makes it a much better choice because the high heats that are used in processing can damage the fat molecules, making them far less healthful.

In this section, oils are used cold, which gives us a greater selection to choose from. Why? Because the most healthful oils—the omega-3 fats you've heard so much about, which are found in fish oil and flaxseed—are actually very unstable, and are easily damaged by heat. That's why you should never use flaxseed oil for cooking and why "deep frying" in canola oil is such a scam. (By the time you have heated the canola oil to the high temperatures needed for frying, it is so damaged that it no longer has any health benefits whatsoever.)

Some of the "healthy" oil blends available, which provide important fatty acids needed for optimal human health, include such brands as Udo's Choice, Omega Balance, Barlean's Essential Woman, and Health from the Sun. Any of the Spectrum cold-pressed organic oils are good, as is flaxseed oil (look for lignan enriched) and, of course, extra-virgin olive oil (though it does not contain any appreciable amount of the desirable omega-3's). Feel free to use these oils interchangeably when oil is called for in any of the snacks.

Yoga for Weight Loss–Friendly Snacks

- Jonny's favorite: handful each of blueberries; cherry tomatoes; 2 ounces Swiss cheese, cubed; half-dozen almonds (optional: sprinkle with oil).
- Raw sliced peppers and tomatoes (optional but recommended: drizzle with oil).
- ½ dozen each of blueberries and cherry tomatoes; 1 ounce almonds (optional: sprinkle with oil).
- ½ prebaked sweet potato—yes, they're delicious cold—with 4 ounces' worth of turkey slices.
- One 6-ounce can sardines; cherry tomatoes.
- Two or three slices of apple smeared with 1 level tablespoon almond or peanut butter.
- 1–2 ounces almonds, pistachio nuts, Brazil nuts, macadamia nuts, pecans, or walnuts.
- Two to three celery sticks smeared with 1 level tablespoon almond or peanut butter.
- A single-serving (3-ounce) can of tuna in water with celery and onion (1 tablespoon of homemade mayo optional, but make it with organic eggs and extra-virgin olive oil—or sprinkle with oil).
- 1 medium tomato, sliced; 2 ounces farmer (or other cheese); sprinkle with oil.

||| 4 turkey slices with sliced tomatoes (optional: sprinkle tomatoes with oil).

||| 2 or 3 leftover beef slices with 3 or 4 slices of tomato (optional: sprinkle tomatoes with oil).

||| 4 ounces of regular yogurt (not the nonfat kind) with 1 ounce almonds.

||| Fresh vegetable juice (if available): good combinations include spinach, parsley, apple, and ginger.

||| Cottage cheese (4 ounces) sprinkled with $1/2$–1 ounce almonds.

Create Your Own Meals

Column A (3–4-ounce portion)	Column B (generous helping)	Column C (starchy carbs—small portion)
Salmon	Spinach	Sweet potato
Tuna	Kale	Corn on the cob
Grouper	Asparagus	Lentils
Mackerel	Artichokes	Beans
Sardines	Bok choy	Basmati rice
Any other fish	Broccoli	Chickpeas
Beef	Collards	Peas
Lamb	Cauliflower	Whole-grain bread (1 slice)
Chicken and turkey		Brussels sprouts
		Carrots
		Cabbage
		Pumpkins
		Squash
		Tomatoes
		Peppers
		Eggplants
		Onions
		Leeks
		Beets
		Cucumbers
		Any other vegetable

Optional Meal Choice

(Can be substituted for any meal on the two-week plan.)

The chart on page 228 lets you mix and match and create your own meals using the basic template of this program. Every meal has one serving of protein, a huge helping of vegetables, and an optional starch in a small portion. You can add a dollop of good fats such as the oils we discussed (keep to one tablespoon), a sliver of avocado, a few nuts, or 1 teaspoon of butter. Choose one item from column A, one from column B, and one from column C.

Soup Recipe

This soup is great alone—or with a salad, for a healthy lunch or dinner meal.

SERVES 6–8

4 green or red peppers, sliced
2 large onions, sliced
6 tomatoes, cubed (or 2 cans of tomatoes)
6 stalks celery, cut in pieces
5 carrots, cut in pieces
2 cups mushrooms, sliced
1 large cabbage (red or green), shredded
8–12 ounces fresh turkey (cooked) or chicken (cooked),
    cut into pieces
1 cup cooked brown rice (you can use Chinese take-out)
Salt, pepper, Chinese seasoning if desired

1. Put all the vegetables in a large soup tureen, pour in enough water to cover all the vegetables, and bring to a boil. Lower flame to a simmer and cook until the vegetables are done (firm but pliable).

2. Add the cooked turkey or chicken and the cooked rice, and stir. Continue to season to taste and check for doneness of the vegetables.

Other Substitutions

There will always be those times when nothing on your program seems to be available, or when you have to just grab something. Here are a couple of options for those situations.

▥ Chinese take-out alternative: Steamed Chicken and Broccoli.

▥ Airport substitutions: Chicken Caesar with extra vegetables, no croutons, and an apple for dessert; meat dish with extra vegetables (no bread, potatoes, or rice) and a single-serving bag of almonds; single-serving size of tuna with celery and carrot sticks and a small apple OR 1 single-size box of raisins.

We hope this chapter has begun a process for you, and that you are now beginning to think differently about food. Changing eating patterns and modifying longstanding habits requires a lot more than just having good information, though. In the next chapter we'll explore some of the critical connections between emotions, food, and habits. For many people, these are connections that a yoga practice helps bring into focus. By understanding these connections and the profound influence they have on your way of relating to food, you will be making a huge step toward substituting new healthful, nourishing habits for old counterproductive ones, and will be on the way to creating a new body and a new way of life.

Chapter Twelve
Food Journaling

"Who are you?" said the caterpillar. Alice replied rather shyly, "I—I hardly know, Sir, just at present— at least I know who I was when I got up this morning, but I think I must have changed several times since then."

—Lewis Carroll, *Alice's Adventures in Wonderland*

If you have weight to lose, there's one thing that's almost for sure: You gained that weight when you weren't looking.

That's right. If you are like most of our clients, your weight was gained almost imperceptibly, over time, without your conscious awareness. Unfortunately, however, the weight you put on without your being aware of it will not come off the same way. It's going to take a heightened awareness and consciousness of everything you put into your body.

In this chapter, we're going to talk about increasing consciousness about your food. Increased consciousness is the single most important tool you have in your arsenal to tackle the problem of excess fat. The entire purpose of this chapter is to keep you more honest, more conscious, and more mindful of your eating.

Trish was a client of Jonny's who, like many people, was frustrated by her inability to lose weight. Convinced she was doing all the right things, she recited a list of the foods she had eaten the previous day: "A small bowl of Grape-Nuts with a little skim milk and a hard-boiled egg, a chicken Caesar salad with some olive oil dressing, some nuts for a snack, and broiled salmon plus vegetables and a potato for dinner. And oh yes, a bowl of berries for dessert." On the face of it this certainly seems like healthful eating, and, with a few modifications, it was.

Then Jonny asked Trish to go to the cupboard and pull out the cereal box. He brought out a food scale and a measuring cup. He then asked Trish to pour the serving size she'd had the day before into a bowl. She did so. He looked at the label, which said "serving size: $\frac{1}{2}$ cup," measured out $\frac{1}{2}$ cup, and poured it into an identical bowl. The bowl Trish had eaten was almost four times the size of the "serving size," a very common occurrence with cereals (as well as pastas, rice, and other starchy carbohydrates). That means that what should have been a 130-calorie serving was in fact a 520-calorie serving! "A little olive oil" could well have turned out to be 3 tablespoons (300 calories), a "potato" could be another 150, "some nuts" could have been anywhere from 180 to 500 calories, and the restaurant-sized portions of chicken and salmon could easily have been 8 ounces each (double what is recommended on our two-week eating plan). All this adds up to a caloric intake of way, way more than the 1,400 or so calories Trish should have been consuming to lose weight. Most of the foods she was eating were good choices, but she was eating much too much of them.

Since most of our eating is unconscious and unmonitored, anything we can do to increase our connectedness with the experience of eating is going to result in more mindful, healthful choices (both in quality of food and in quantity). This mindfulness nearly always leads to more weight loss, not to mention a healthier attitude toward food and nourishment. This chapter will give you some valuable tools to create that sense of connectedness to your own eating habits, helping to make them less automatic and unconscious, and enabling you to become more fully present in the nourishing of your body.

The Food Journal

As noted in Chapter 2, research indicates that there are two activities that best predict success in keeping weight off. One of them is exercise; the other is keeping a food journal. It's impossible to overstate how important the journal is to the success of the program. Here's why: Most people have no idea how many calories they eat every day. Most of our food is consumed unconsciously—on the run, while watching television, at fast-food restaurants, or from take-out establishments. While we may have some vague idea that we are eating "too much" or "the wrong things," we don't have real clarity about how much is too much, or what things are wrong for us and why. So we go on doing what we're doing without a real sense of purpose or vision for what our bodies truly need.

Over time, a food journal allows you to make the connection between what you eat and what your body really needs. It will help you distinguish what your body needs from what your mind wants, and, as you progress, will make those two things more alike. It will help connect you to the source of your food, to the activity of eating, to the processes involved in bringing it to your table. In much the same way as a yoga pose makes you more aware of your body, the food journal makes you more aware of the processes that sustain that body over time. If you keep your journal diligently, it will almost certainly help you lose weight.

How Do I Do It?

The food journal works like this: Every day you're going to keep track of exactly what you eat and drink, and when. Buy a notebook—a journal of your own that you can keep with you at all times.

Use the sample pages in this chapter as a guide. At the end of each meal, write down what you've eaten. It's better if you do it meal by meal rather than trying to reconstruct your meals at the end of the day. Be scrupulously honest. Try to estimate the portion size as much as possible. Write down the time of day that you eat. Take note of your energy level. Were you tired after a meal, or were you energized? What was the connection between what you ate and how you felt? Did you get "foggy," or did you feel "sharper"? What about the relationship between how many hours you slept and how hungry you were?

Rate your level of hunger after each meal. Did you feel satisfied? Full? Stuffed? Still hungry? Was there a relationship between what you ate and how hungry you were afterwards? (For example, did you tend to feel more satisfied if your meal contained meat?) Notice that and write it down. How many hours on average do you spend between feedings? When did your energy tend to sag during the day, and can you find any relationship between your energy level and what you're eating?

Mary was a client of Jonny's who kept the food journal scrupulously and discovered a number of surprising facts. She had been under the impression that she was consuming about 1,300 calories a day, but her totals added up to well over 1,750. Since she was five-foot-three and weighed 150 pounds when she started the program, an intake this high was not going to produce her weight loss goal. Second, her protein intake was only about 10 percent of her diet. Since she was trying to eat "low-fat," this left the bulk of her calories coming from carbohydrates. She noticed that she was constantly tired, especially in the afternoons and late mornings, and that she often didn't have energy for her workouts. When she modified her diet to contain protein at every meal, reduced her carbohydrate intake from processed carbs such as pasta, bread, and cereals, increased her fruits and vegetables, and added back the good fats discussed in this book (olive oil, avocado, nuts, seeds, butter, and flaxseed oil) she noticed that she was no longer as tired, didn't have "energy crashes" midmorning and midafternoon, was able to sustain exercise longer, and began to sleep better. Her cravings slowly disappeared and her meals began leaving her feeling satisfied for several hours or more. Gradually she began to lose weight, and as of this writing is down to 130, just 10 pounds away from her goal.

Mary—like many of our clients who have had similar results—is sure that these results would not have been achieved had she not incorporated the food journal into her life. She feels it gave her the ability to look fearlessly and honestly at what she was really doing with food, and that the information she got from journaling allowed her to make conscious, mindful changes that led to her success.

Sample Layouts

Here's a sample of how you might lay out a page in your food journal:

Number of hours slept last night

_____

Quality of my sleep: Poor / Fair / Average / Good / Excellent

Time:

_____

Food eaten:

_____

_____

_____

_____

After eating I feel: Still hungry / Somewhat hungry / Not hungry / Full / Stuffed

Energy level: Very Low / Low / Average / High / Very High

Time:

_____

Food eaten:

_____

_____

_____

_____

After eating I feel: Still hungry / Somewhat hungry / Not hungry / Full / Stuffed

Energy level: Very Low / Low / Average / High / Very High

Time:

Food eaten:

After eating I feel: Still hungry / Somewhat hungry / Not hungry / Full / Stuffed

Energy level: Very Low / Low / Average / High / Very High

Making the Connections

When you keep records like these for at least a few days, you will probably notice a number of things. First, the very fact that you are writing down what you are eating causes you to pay more attention to what's going into your body. Second, the process causes you to be more observant; you may find that you are actually noticing portion sizes in a way that you weren't before. Third, you may find yourself making healthier choices simply because you don't want to have to write down the amount of junk that you would otherwise be consuming. A number of our clients actually changed the way they were eating because they said they would have been too embarrassed to show us their journals if they kept on eating the way they had been before starting the journal!

It would be great if you set up your journal so that you had a place to note things like your mood and your energy. You may begin to notice connections between what you eat and how you feel. You may also begin to notice connections between what you are feeling and what you choose to eat. Remember, yoga is about observation and truth as much as it is about anything else. Approach your food journal with an attitude of consciousness and peacefulness. Don't judge, just observe.

Try the food journal for at least a week. After completing the week of journaling, please answer the following questions in your journal, or right here in the book if you like.

What have I noticed that's true for me after a week of food journaling?

_____

_____

_____

_____

_____

What changes do I need to make to be where I want to be?

_____

_____

_____

_____

_____

What actions am I going to take right now to make this happen?

1. _____

2. _____

3. _____

4. _____

Accelerated Progress

We've developed some exercises to increase your ability to connect with your food even more. Think of this section as a kind of "yoga for eating"; we want you to raise your consciousness not only of the eating process, but of the cooking, preparing, and gathering of food as well.

Do each of these exercises at least once (more if you like), or repeat them any time you feel you are beginning to get disconnected from the process of eating.

The Chocolate Trip

Go to the store to buy some chocolate. (Don't use just any chocolate you have lying around—you want this exercise to be special!) You should get the best, richest, most expensive kind you can find, but the smallest amount possible. Godiva is a good choice. Try to choose chocolate that has a variety of layers or textures, though this is not necessary.

Carve out a one-inch-square piece of the chocolate and put the rest away. If it comes premade in single bite-size pieces, use one of those. Whatever one you choose, let it be the perfect piece.

Find a comfortable place where you can be alone for 10 minutes or so. Get into your yoga frame of mind. Sit comfortably on the floor. You can put on soft meditative music in the background, though this is not necessary. Light some incense if you like. Make the space yours.

Now take the chocolate and hold it up to your eyes at a comfortable level. Look at it. Feel yourself becoming more observant. What are some things you never noticed about chocolate before? How deep is the color? How many layers are there? Imagine what it might be like if you were a Lilliputian traveler (thumb-sized people from *Gulliver's Travels*) and were climbing up a mound of just this kind of chocolate. What would it feel like under your hands and feet? What would it feel like to climb inside? What would it smell like?

Notice what your senses are doing and saying.

Now take a small bite of the chocolate. Hold it in your mouth. Put it under your tongue. Imagine the receptors in your tongue. What are they saying? What does it feel like? What does it really taste like before you swallow it? Is it bitter? Sweet? Bittersweet? See how many textures and tastes you can discern. Roll it around in your mouth. Imagine the juices of your mouth working on the chocolate, melting it away into warm liquid. What does that look like? What does it taste like?

Finally, swallow the chocolate. Feel it journeying down your throat. What is the sensation? What is the aftertaste?

Look at the remaining chocolate. Imagine the sensation you just had of eating it. Imagine all that sensation contained as unexpressed energy inside the chocolate. Consider how that energy is released when you pop the remaining amount in your mouth. Feel how the warmth of your mouth liberates the energy contained in the chocolate and creates the sensation that you're feeling as you roll it around your tongue. Finally, swallow the remaining liquid.

How would you describe the experience to a stranger who had never tasted chocolate?

Repeat the exercise with a strawberry.

The Television Exercise

Studies have shown a relationship between overeating and television watching.

There is a direct correlation between obesity and the number of hours of television watched. We don't know for sure why this is. One theory is the sheer numbers of commercials for food that the average television viewer sees. (By one estimation, the average American will be exposed to 350,000 television commercials by the time he reaches voting age, 80 percent of them for high-calorie junk food.) Another theory is that when you sit in front of the television for up to five hours a day, that's five hours a day that you are not doing physical activity. A third theory is that watching television promotes the kind of unconscious eating and nibbling that is the enemy of weight loss programs of all types, everywhere.

No matter which theory is correct—to be sure, all of them may be partially right—the bottom line remains the same: Television and food are a lethal combination if you're trying to lose weight and if you're trying to eat mindfully.

In the Television Exercise you're going to eat at least one meal a day completely away from the television. You can make this exercise most meaningful if you choose a meal when you would normally watch television, such as dinner. During this exercise, you don't even want to have the TV going in the background. If you are accustomed to eating every meal with the television on, start by weaning yourself off one meal at a time. The idea is to get to the point at which you don't eat any meals in front of the television.

The Silence Exercise

Eat an entire meal in silence. Try to bring some of the consciousness from the chocolate (or strawberry) exercise into the experience. Be aware of every bite. Look at your food. Chew thoroughly. Try putting the fork down between bites. Don't rush. What did you notice? Write it down in your journal!

Molly's Gratitude Exercise

Take yourself through a gratitude checklist with every meal. You can think of this as a kind of "grace."

1. Thank the universe for the food you are about to eat.

2. Thank those responsible for cooking and preparing it (especially if it is you).

3. Thank those responsible for growing it and harvesting it and preparing it for sale at the store.

4. If your food was once a living animal or fish, thank it for giving its life so that you may be nourished and so that the chain of life may continue on.

5. Be aware of the energy that created the conditions under which your food was grown or harvested—the sun, the moon, and the earth.

Begin to notice when your foods are not "real" foods. As you begin to be more aware of the life force in your food, you will also become more aware of when you are eating dead, prepackaged, and processed food products, as opposed to real foods with life energy. Try to shift more and more toward real foods. They will not only nourish and sustain you better, but they will fill you up and create metabolic conditions more likely to result in your achieving your weight loss goals.

Chapter Thirteen
Calories and Consciousness

*We shall not cease from
   exploration
And the end of all our
   exploring
Will be to arrive where
   we started
And know the place for
   the first time.*

—T. S. Eliot

The food journal you began in Chapter 12 is the first step in your journey to increased mindfulness and consciousness about food, which in turn will lead you to a heightened awareness of what you need to do to control and manage your weight for the rest of your life. Just as the asanas in the first part of the book will help you to strengthen and tone your body for maximum fat-burning effectiveness, the techniques in this part of the book will help you to gain control of your eating and to design an eating program for yourself that will support you in having the body you want and deserve.

Three Steps Toward Fat-Melting Success

There are three steps in our eating program:

1. Observe
2. Evaluate
3. Correct

Writing in your journal is just the first step. It's the "truth-telling" part of the exercise. It's easy to see, however, that just telling the truth about what you're eating—the "observation" step—is not enough to cause fat to melt off your body. (We can all imagine a scenario in which someone eats six junk-food meals a day and simply records every bite in the journal.) To make meaningful changes, we need to evaluate what we're eating (the second step) and then, if necessary, make some corrections (the third step).

The journal writing will give you a baseline—an accurate picture of what you are actually doing when it comes to food. Now let's see if we can lay down some general guidelines against which to evaluate and correct your current diet.

Guideline Number One: Calories

To get an estimate of the number of calories you should be consuming, add a zero to the weight you would like to be. That will give you a good approximation of the number of calories you should be consuming during the weight loss phase. For example, if you currently weigh 180 pounds but are aiming to go down to 130, your target caloric intake should be about 1,300 calories until you've lost the weight. But you might start at a more reasonable goal of 150 or 160 pounds and bring your caloric intake down less drastically. While every case is going to be different, the majority of weight loss programs for women will range from 1,250 to 1,500 calories per day, and the majority of weight loss programs for men will range from 1,500 to 2,000 calories. You should never go below 1,000 calories a day. We don't even like the idea of anyone going below 1,250. It is virtually impossible to get complete nutrition at the 1,000-calorie mark, and even flirting with a caloric intake this low is counterproductive from a weight loss point of view for reasons that will be made clear shortly.

Molly Fox's Yoga Weight Loss Program allows about 1,300 to 1,600 calories per day; if you follow the plan and feel it's too much food, you can bring it down if you need to by either eliminating the snacks or slightly reducing the portions, but it is unlikely that you'll have to do this. If, on the other hand, you're exercising a lot—and are very active and feel you need a bit more food—just up the portions slightly or have another snack. Remember, your biochemistry is uniquely yours; no one will respond exactly like you, and you need to honor this individuality in developing the program that works for you.

Buying an inexpensive calorie counter would be a good purchase at this point, simply as an educational tool. There are dozens available in every bookstore, usually for no more than a few dollars. Your purpose is not to be obsessive about calorie counting, but to educate yourself as to what is really going into your body so that you can evaluate and correct as needed.

Don't worry—you won't need to use the calorie counter for the rest of your life. It's simply a tool to help you better understand the difference between what you are currently consuming and what you actually need. Many of our clients find using the calorie counter to be both interesting and an eye-opener. It can also be fun. It doesn't have to be tedious. Make a game of it. See if you can guess the number of calories and amount of carbohydrate, fat, or protein in a given food and then test yourself by checking in the book. Were you way off? Most people are. Make sure to attend carefully to the portion size to get an accurate picture of what's going on.

A second item to consider buying at this point is a food scale. Much like the calorie counter, it can be an amazing help to the conscious eater. The thing that really convinced Jonny of the value of the food scale was his experience with pasta. When he first measured out 2 ounces of uncooked spaghetti on the scale to see what a 210-calorie "portion" really looked like, it was a revelation. When cooked, this portion didn't look like any portion any of us had seen in a restaurant in the last 10 years, nor did it resemble the portion size most of us had seen served at friends' houses. It's easy to see why pasta gets such a bad rap; in addition to being high glycemic (it converts to sugar in the body very quickly, causing fat storage hormones to go into full gear), it is maddeningly easy to overeat.

Use the scale to measure out portion sizes as suggested on the labels so that you can increase your consciousness about how much you're eating. It's particularly good for measuring ounces of protein, and will quickly give you a clear idea of what a 3- or 4-ounce serving of meat (or chicken or fish) looks like so that you can better estimate what you're eating when you eat at restaurants. After using the food scale for a short while, you may find yourself cutting restaurant portions in half and, more often than not, asking for "doggy bags."

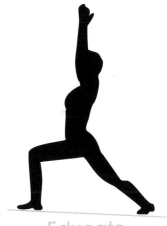

Educate yourself **as to what is really going into your body.**

Guideline Number Two: Protein

To get a general idea of how much protein you need, divide your goal weight by 10. That's the minimum number of ounces of protein you should be getting on a daily basis. For example, if your goal weight is 150 pounds, you should be getting at least 15 ounces of protein each day; if your goal weight is 130 pounds, you should be getting at least 13 ounces a day. Ideally that should be divided evenly among all your meals, but as a practical matter that may not be possible. If it isn't, try to get some protein at every meal or snack and keep the distribution as even as is reasonably possible. For example, the person with the goal of at least 13 ounces a day who was eating four times a day (three meals and one snack) might choose 4 ounces at each of three meals and 2 ounces at her snack; if she was eating five times a day (three meals and two snacks), she might choose $3\frac{1}{2}$ to 4 ounces at each of three meals and 1 to 2 ounces per snack. If you are using a protein powder as a protein source, you should count 7 grams as 1 ounce of meat; thus a typical 20-gram serving scoop of protein powder is roughly the equivalent of 3 ounces of cooked meat.

A Note about Vegetarianism

You will notice that in the two-week eating plan (Chapter 11), as well as in the general guidelines for eating, there is a lot of emphasis on animal foods like chicken, turkey, lean meat, and eggs (as well as fish, which can be eaten by some people who still consider themselves, for the most part, vegetarians). Since yoga is traditionally associated with a vegetarian lifestyle, this emphasis on animal protein probably deserves a little explanation.

Jonny believes firmly that the diet we were designed to eat—the one that sustained and nourished the human genus for 2.4 million years, *Homo erectus* for 1.8 million, and *Homo sapiens* for at least the past 130,000 years—was composed of foods we could hunt, fish, gather, pluck, and, much later, grow. This is the hunter-gatherer diet, and, although there is evidence that it varied depending on the region, it was always made up of meat or fish plus vegetation. Sweets were infrequent treats, and processed food was, of course, unknown. Agriculture didn't come into existence until 10,000 years ago, so for the most part we did not have grains, domestic farm animals, or cultivated crops until then, and had to survive on what we could catch or find.

A full discussion of the enormous evidence for the value of what is sometimes called a "Paleolithic" or "caveman" diet is beyond the scope of this book, though Jonny has written about it elsewhere. The bottom line is that we—humankind—seem to fare best on a native diet which, like it or not, has always included animal products. This does not mean that you cannot lose weight and be healthy if you are a vegetarian. You certainly can. But it does mean that, vegetarian or not, you must pay particular attention to the presence and quality of protein in your diet, as well as good-quality fats. A diet too high in carbohydrates—particularly the processed, manufactured kinds that constitute the overwhelming majority of the carbohydrates we eat in modern society—is a huge obstacle to weight loss for many people (perhaps you are among them). This is why this program emphasizes protein, good fats, vegetables, a certain amount of fruit, and a reduced contribution from starchy carbs like rice, potatoes, bread, pasta, and cereals.

The problem is compounded by what nutritionists sometimes refer to as "Twinkie vegetarians." Jonny has frequently seen clients who come in thinking that they are eating a healthful diet because they don't eat meat. They proudly proclaim they are vegetarians. Yet their food journals show a tremendous preponderance of cereals, pastas, cakes, cookies, snack foods, macaroni and cheese, breads, and soft drinks. There is absolutely nothing healthful about this kind of diet, and it is a complete disaster for weight loss. Yet it is, technically, a "vegetarian" diet. The moral of the story: Don't fall for the idea that simply because a diet is vegetarian it is necessarily healthful.

If you want to follow Molly Fox's Yoga Weight Loss Program from a vegetarian perspective, you must be very conscious of getting high-quality protein and fats from nonanimal sources if this is your preference. If you are the kind of vegetarian who eats eggs and fish, you will have no problem whatsoever. Between those two wonderful foods plus protein powders made from soy or whey, you will be set. If you don't eat those foods, you will have to get your protein from soy protein powders, tofu, and other nonanimal sources. An excellent cookbook for this approach is *The Schwarzbein Principle Vegetarian Cookbook,* by Diana Schwarzbein, M.D.

Guideline Number Three: Fat

We don't recommend counting fat grams obsessively. America has become far too obsessed with fat-reducing diets, and this wrong-headed emphasis has resulted in consumption of foods that are much too high in starch, grains, sugar, and processed food, and too low in fiber and healthful fats like the omega-3's found in fish. We prefer that you concentrate on the quality of fat in your diet rather than the absolute amount. Your fat should come from whole, natural foods like fish, avocados, nuts, nut butters, butter, and olive oil. You should avoid margarines, fried foods, and anything that says "hydrogenated" on the label, which will include most baked goods, pastries, cookies, crackers, and snack cakes, as well as many processed foods.

It's perfectly acceptable not to count fat grams and to simply allow each meal to contain a reasonable amount of healthful fat (approximately one-third of the calories in any given meal). You don't have to do any further calculation. But for those who feel more comfortable with a more precise guideline for fat intake, here's how to estimate it:

- Start with the first three digits of your total calorie intake. (For example, if your daily caloric goal is 1,300 calories, the first three digits would be 130.)
- Multiply that number by 3. (For example, 130 × 3 = 390.)
- Divide that number by 9 and round off the answer. (For example, 390 / 9 = 43.)

That will be the approximate number of grams of fat you should have in your daily diet.

Once again, as with protein, the bull's-eye is to distribute that fat evenly among at least four feedings. For example, in the above example of a 1,300-calorie day with 43 grams of fat, we would be shooting for approximately 11 grams of fat per meal or feeding. However, it's perfectly acceptable to break it up differently, as long as you adhere to the spirit of the idea of consuming fat (and protein) at every meal rather than "saving up" the day's "allowance" for one big splurge. So, for example, a person eating 1,300 calories a day and eating three meals and one snack might have 12 grams of fat per meal and 7 grams of fat in her snack; a person eating 1,300 calories a day and eating three meals and two snacks might have 10 grams of fat per meal and 7 grams per snack.

Guideline Number Four: Carbohydrates

The rest of your food should be carbohydrates. Remember, all carbohydrates are not "bad." There has been a tendency in the diet establishment to link all carbohydrates together as if they are one homogeneous group of equal value (or equal danger). They are not. Candy bars are carbohydrates, but so is cauliflower; pasta and bread are carbohydrates, but so are apples and Brussels sprouts. The trick here is to fill your plate with unprocessed carbohydrates (the kind that doesn't come in packages!). This means loading up your plate with vegetables, legumes (beans), and some fruit (preferably berries).

Although fruit is one of the "good" carbohydrates, we recommend that for weight loss purposes you keep your fruit servings to two a day and get the rest of your "fruits and vegetables" servings from vegetables. This is due to the higher sugar content of fruit. Higher sugar can trigger higher levels of the hormone insulin in sensitive people (at least one-quarter of the population), which can set in motion fat-storing metabolic processes in your body and make it fiendishly difficult to lose weight. We want to keep the sugar intake low. Even though the sugar in fruit is a natural, the body still "sees" it as sugar and treats it accordingly.

Some fruits are higher in sugar than others (such as ripe bananas and tropical fruits) and others (such as berries) are much lower. For this reason, we recommend that you get your fruit servings from berries whenever possible. Raspberries, strawberries, blueberries, and blackberries are all superb choices. Other lower-sugar fruits include apples, apricots, plums, and cherries.

Some of the carbohydrates on your menu can be from starch, but we recommend that you keep the starchy carbohydrates to a minimum and choose carefully from low-glycemic starches, such as oatmeal, sweet potatoes, and beans instead of commercial pastas and breads. Low-glycemic, you will recall, refers to the fact that these foods convert to sugar in the body at a lower speed than high-glycemic foods, such as pastas and breads. (For a fuller discussion of high- and low-glycemic foods, see Chapter 10). The occasional slice of whole grain bread is fine, but eating sandwiches regularly will put you well over our limits for daily intake of starchy grains. If you can cut bread and pasta out altogether, that would not be a bad thing. At the very least, make them occasional treats rather than a part of your daily intake.

A Simplified Plan

If you would prefer not to compute the amount of protein, carbohydrate, and fat in each meal, here's a simpler way to do it. Simply take your plate and mentally divide it into thirds. Now don't overfill it—remember to keep an eye on portion size. Fill one-third with protein foods (chicken, fish, tofu, meat, eggs). Fill the remaining two-thirds with vegetables (or leave some room for berries). Once in a while some of that space for vegetables can be partly filled with a starch like sweet potatoes or oatmeal. Add a dollop of healthy fat to the mix, either as a dressing (olive oil), part of the meal (fish like salmon), or seasoning (a little butter melted over vegetables or oatmeal). Voilà. A perfect meal—and you never have to count calories, fat grams, protein, or carbohydrate.

Does Calorie Reduction Always Lead to Weight Loss?

You may remember that earlier we urged you never to reduce calories below 1,000 a day, and to avoid going lower than 1,250. Why would we make this recommendation when it seems clear that reducing calories leads to weight loss? Wouldn't it make sense that the lower you go, the more weight you lose?

Like most things, the answer is more complicated than it seems. On the surface, yes, if you reduce calories enough, you will at first lose weight. However, there are several reasons why this is an incomplete approach.

Number one, it doesn't address the nature of those calories, so from a purely health perspective, the calories-is-all theory is very weak; it reduces foods as complicated and different as a Snickers bar and a plate of cauliflower to nothing more than their caloric content. That would be like reducing a human being to simply the amount of money he or she earns without factoring in any other considerations.

Number two, when you eat food you stimulate hormones. If the amount of food is too little, you stimulate cortisol and adrenaline, which ultimately leads to muscle breakdown and the reduction of metabolic rate (not good). If you eat too much, you stimulate insulin, which ultimately leads to fat storage (also not good). If your carbohydrate or sugar intake is too great, the same thing happens as when you eat too much food—both your blood sugar and your insulin levels rise, and you will be in full-tilt "fat storage" mode. On the other hand, if your carbohydrate intake is much too low, you risk stimulating more cortisol. So while a lower calorie intake is definitely a good thing up to a point, your calorie intake should never go too low. You should be concentrating on the right kind of calories rather than just the total amount. That means adequate fat and protein at every meal and good, real-food carbohydrates. Divide that caloric intake into small meals and eat them every three or four hours, and you'll be fine. Your weight loss might be a bit slower than drastic caloric reduction, but it will last longer and be more permanent, and it will really be fat that you're losing, not muscle mass. You'll also be healthier.

All this adds up to one thing: more mindful eating. If you'll recall, what distinguishes this eating program from the others you may have seen is that while it does indeed talk about calories, fat, protein, and carbohydrates, it does so not for the purpose of giving you an absolute prescription to follow, but rather, to increase your consciousness about food. You need to know exactly what is going into your body and how it affects your mood, your energy, and of course, your weight, before you are going to be able to make any meaningful changes. Remember: Observe, evaluate, and then correct. Yoga is about observation of your inner world, and a big part of that inner world is the way you think and feel—whether consciously or unconsciously—about food.

In Chapter 12 we did some exercises to help you move some of that unconscious thinking about food into your consciousness, allowing you to look at it truthfully and fearlessly and without judgment. In the next chapter we're going to help you reprogram yourself to hold positive ideas and associations about eating, losing weight, and exercising.

It is from this space of consciousness and mindfulness that you will most effectively be able to make the changes you need to make to have a body that you can love, appreciate, and live in happily.

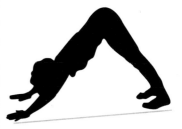

Remember: Observe, evaluate, and then correct.

Chapter Fourteen
Weight Management with
Self-Hypnosis: Visualizations

Whether you think you
can or think you can't,
you are right.

—Henry Ford

Self-hypnosis is a powerful tool for clarifying your weight management goals, visualizing your desired outcome, and releasing any
blocks you may be experiencing on the way there. Alone, or combined with Molly Fox's Yoga Weight Loss Program, a regular practice
of self-hypnosis can bring about a profound sense of well-being.

I first became interested in using self-hypnosis as a tool for my
weight loss clients because my sister Katie had used the technique
quite successfully in her own practice and in her own life, with
amazing results. Here is Katie's story in her own words.

Katie's Story

*When I decided, deep within my heart, that I wanted to allow my
body to return to a healthy weight, I chose to use a combination of
self-hypnosis and yoga. Both have been part of my life for many years
now, but using these tools consciously for weight release was an
intriguing opportunity.*

*Conceptually, the process was one of release and ease, rather
than struggle and deprivation. During my practice, I would hold the
intention of my body feeling light, flexible, and strong. I used my
breath and self-hypnosis tools to bring myself into a more present
and receptive state, where I could visualize my body letting go of
restrictions, limitations, and excess weight. Practice became even*

more joyful, and new discoveries about each pose came easily to me. My day-to-day choices about food were less angst-ridden, as my deep desire to feel lighter and better drove me to focus on what I could eat, not what I couldn't. I discovered a new joy from being fully present and in my body.

I lost 15 pounds and have reached a healthy, comfortable weight that I would like to maintain. Maintenance has new challenges, but I am ready and willing to learn about how to stay here. Since my weight loss journey, my life has become more open, one of possibility and promise, and I am truly "traveling light."

Self-Hypnosis and Weight Management

All hypnosis is really self-hypnosis, and is merely a state of deep physical relaxation and focused awareness, combined with visualizations and specific statements we make to ourselves. Moving into a hypnotic trance is something we all do easily and perhaps even without realizing it. For example, you're in a form of a hypnotic state when you are driving, unconsciously turning the wheel, knowing instinctively how to get home while thinking of your to-do list. Similarly, when you are engrossed in a fabulous book, or a fascinating conversation—and you're only vaguely aware of what's happening around you—you're in a kind of a trance. Self-hypnosis brings about a state that we can arrive at readily and easily and, with a little practice, use to bring about positive change.

The process of releasing unwanted weight through relaxation and visualization is based on the premise that weight management is about expansion, not contraction. It's not based on deprivation, strict diets, or self-judgment. In fact, as we discover our true selves and the love we can experience for ourselves by getting in touch with our deeper or unconscious mind, we find we're focusing on what we can have, and on the loving relationships we do have. The process of discovering optimal physical health therefore becomes a pleasant one. As we expand and discover possibility, we create more space in our worlds and in our bodies for what makes us truly happy, and our bodies respond by releasing weight. We then come from a place of expecting to be light and happy with our bodies, and our new, health-promoting beliefs and behaviors grow out of this state of mind.

To arrange a self-hypnosis session for yourself, all you need is some free time, a quiet place, and, ideally, a self-hypnosis tape. We can help you make your own personalized tape. If you follow our instructions, you will be able to use it to enjoy a relaxing and productive self-hypnosis session anytime you want. Before you start, make sure you read through How to Make Your Own Self-Hypnosis Tape (later in this chapter) so you can get an idea of what you'll be doing.

Here is the basic format for your self-hypnosis session.

Take Your Time

First, you need to set aside some free time, turn off the phones and any other distractions, and tell your family you're going to be taking some personal time. You'll want to be certain you won't be disturbed.

Find Your Space

Next, find your comfortable place to relax. Your sacred space is a great choice. It's best if you're sitting up in a chair, but you can also recline. Make sure you're wearing comfortable clothing so you can really relax and let go.

Play Your Self-Hypnosis Tape

Once you've prepared the tape based on our directions in How to Make Your Own Self-Hypnosis Tape, all you have to do is relax and listen to your own voice. You can use headphones if you like.

Follow Up with Tools for Success

Once you have completed your session, it's especially good to follow up immediately with an activity to jell your suggestions in your mind and body. Here are a few ideas for activities to complement and reinforce self-hypnosis after a session.

1. Practice a few yoga poses of your choice.

2. Journal, draw, or dance.

3. Go for a walk outside and breathe fresh air.

4. Talk with a friend.

5. Take a bath.

Using your own tape and designing your own self-hypnosis session can bring about exciting changes in your body, your mind, and in your life. Be creative and make up new self-suggestions as you go along, to give yourself some variety. Or add a little soothing music to the background. You can always record new tapes.

Through this self-hypnosis program you can rediscover the pleasure of being in your body. You'll probably respect it more and want to take care of it better to get healthier. You will learn to accept that ebb and flow in our bodies is normal, and perhaps even essential to life. This fluctuation can be a source of comfort as you learn flexibility and gentleness toward yourself about the food you eat, your level of activity, and the beliefs you hold about yourself and your body. In this way, you will be well on the road to making lasting lifestyle changes that you can truly live with.

How to Make Your Own Self-Hypnosis Tape

To make your own self-hypnosis tape, you will record the script we've prepared for you, along with self-suggestions you have designed for yourself. Here are the steps for preparing your self-suggestions.

Writing Your Own Script

1. Create your image goal.

First, you need to get out a pen and paper and do a little writing. A few paragraphs are plenty. Answer the following questions in as much detail as you can.

- How do you feel about your body right now, today? When you look in the mirror, what do you see?
- If you would like that to change, how would you like to feel about your body instead?
- Can you remember feeling that way before? When?
- Begin to form a picture in your mind of you with the healthiest body you can imagine for yourself, and describe how you look.

2. Set your intention.

Review your answers to the above questions, then use those answers to begin to define your overall goal for your health and weight. This could be specific, as in wanting to fit into a specific size, or more general, as in wanting to have more energy and to enjoy life more. Write it down in one sentence below.

Example: My goal is to have a healthy and toned body, and to be able to exercise vigorously for half an hour.

My goal is to:

_____

_____

Now rewrite this goal as if you are talking to yourself, and it has already happened. We'll call this sentence "your intention."

Example: You have a healthy and toned body, and you easily exercise vigorously for half an hour.

Your intention:

_____

_____

_____

_____

This intention is part of the script you will record later.

3. Script your self-suggestions.

BELIEFS: Think about specific beliefs you would like to have to reach this goal. For example, a new belief could be that you love and accept your body unconditionally. Write down a few below:

_____

_____

Now, write these new beliefs as if you're talking to yourself. Be positive.

Examples of self-suggestions for new beliefs:

- Anytime you need to feel good about your body, you'll remember the picture of yourself in the healthiest body you can imagine, and you'll be filled with pride and love.
- My body is beautiful, full of life, and energetic.

Your belief self-suggestions:

_____

_____

4. Behaviors

Think about specific behaviors that you know are preventing you from reaching your goal, and that you would like to change. For example, it might be that you would like to stop eating a big piece of chocolate when you crave it, and eat small amounts of chocolate or even a healthful snack alternative instead.

Write down a few of those behaviors here:

_____

_____

_____

_____

_____

Now, write down new behaviors to replace your current ones. Write them as if you're talking to yourself. Keep your language positive!

Examples of self-suggestions for new behaviors:

- Any time you crave chocolate, you will reach for a healthful snack instead, such as an apple.
- When you are eating a meal, you will chew slowly, and will stop eating as soon as you are satisfied.

Your behavior self-suggestions:

_____

_____

_____

_____

_____

_____

Recording Your Tape

You now have all the personalized information you need to record your tape. You will add them to the self-hypnosis scripts below.

The following is the order for recording your scripts—it's very important to follow this exactly! As you read and record, flow easily from one script to the next so it seems like one complete script.

- Relaxation Script
- Positive Visualization Script
- Your Personalized Scripts:
  a. Your intention
  b. Your belief self-suggestions
  c. Your behavior self-suggestions
- Coming Up Script

Recording Tips

1. Record your scripts either in your own voice, or have someone else record them, if you find their voice to be soothing.
2. Speak slowly, but clearly, and in a gentle, "hypnotic" voice. Imagine you are reading a book to a child.
3. Allow plenty of time at the indicated pauses (don't read "pause"). When you are relaxed, you'll appreciate having that time.

Now, let's begin recording your tape.

Sit back . . . Relax . . . Close your eyes . . . Begin to become aware of your breathing . . . (pause) As you take each breath slowly, you will become more and more deeply relaxed and comfortable . . . (pause) Begin to feel every part of your body just relaxing . . . just relax . . . now.

Take a few moments to become aware of your body . . . notice how it feels . . . and if you are noticing any places of tension . . . or relaxation. . . . Listen to any sounds around you, letting yourself experience . . . whatever reaches your senses. . . . Be in your body and relax completely . . . just relaxing now. Good.

Now take three deep breaths . . . inhaling so that your body fills with fresh air . . . feeling yourself relax completely as you exhale . . . completely . . . (pause) Continuing to relax . . . going deeper . . . waiting patiently for your body to take its next breath after your completed exhale . . . (pause) Continue relaxing . . . observing your breathing until you can comfortably wait for at least three seconds after exhaling completely and before taking the next inhale . . . (long pause)

In a moment, I will mention parts of your body, and when I mention those parts of your body, you will feel them relax easily and comfortably . . . Starting at your head, you will progressively tense, then relax each part of your body. Inhaling as you tense the body part, then relaxing even more deeply as you exhale completely.

Feel your jaw, then tense it . . . tense your entire face, just really screw it up . . . hold for five counts: 1 . . . 2 . . . 3 . . . 4 . . . 5, and exhaling completely, relax your jaw . . . completely. Now tense all the skin on your scalp, hold it for five seconds, and then relax . . . completely. Become aware of your eyes, and the darkness you see behind your closed eyelids. Now shut your eyes really tight, then relax them and feel the heaviness in your eyelids. A heaviness . . . coming over your very, very relaxed eyelids. Feeling your neck— front, back, and sides of your neck . . . tense your shoulders into your neck and really feel that tension release when you exhale . . . exhaling now . . . neck and shoulders heavy and completely relaxed. Aware of your upper back and chest . . . tensing that area, then relaxing in completely as your exhale deeply and completely . . . Making fists as you inhale again . . . and tensing your arms completely . . . now letting go completely . . . hands and arms deeply relaxed now . . . aware of your hips and buttocks . . . tensing them so much you almost lift off . . . now exhale and relax your hips and buttocks completely. So relaxed now. Now . . . inhaling and tensing your legs and feet . . . pointing your toes . . . now . . . exhale and relaxing your legs and feet completely. Taking one full inhale again throughout your body . . . exhaling and feeling your whole body relax even deeper as you exhale completely. Just like a balloon that has lost all of its air. So very relaxed now . . . Feeling your eyelids again . . . how heavy and relaxed they are . . . And, only when you are sure you cannot open them, . . . try to open your eyes and see how they just become even heavier . . . now stop trying and notice how relaxed you are now . . . (pause)

Now you will take yourself to even deeper levels of relaxation, where you can really make positive changes in your life and . . . bring about a sense of well-being.

With your eyes closed, imagine a screen with 10 numbers on it: 10 going down to 1. The numbers will light up as they represent your level of relaxation. You are now at 10, and as I count down to 1, you will become much more relaxed with every number I count . . . 10 . . . going down . . . 9 . . . seeing the number 9 lighting up now . . . 8 . . . more relaxed . . . 7 . . . deeper down . . . 6 . . . very relaxed . . . 5 . . . relaxing even more now . . . 4 . . . 3 . . . 2 . . . too relaxed to care anymore . . . and . . . 1 . . . Veeerrrrry . . . deeply . . . relaxed . . . now. Very good.

Positive Visualization Script

Because you are now so relaxed and peaceful, you know you can be successful in anything you want, and can achieve any goal you set for yourself. Imagine yourself in a place where you can be completely relaxed and completely yourself. It could be someplace you've been before, or someplace you'd like to go. It could even be an imaginary place. You're feeling great and enjoying life. See yourself as your ideal self. Let the scene come in clearly . . . Let it be what it is and enter into the scene completely . . . Look around you, smell the smells, and experience this place fully. You might be in your body, or you might be looking at yourself. Either is just fine. Count from 1 to 5 and let the scene play out, feeling relaxed and completely yourself. Noticing how wonderful and healthy you are. 1 . . . 2 . . . 3 . . . 4 . . . 5.

Now keep that wonderful feeling with you and let that scene fade away. Now imagine yourself sitting in a chair at a table, having a meal. It might be alone or with family or friends. You are enjoying the food—it's healthful and satisfying. You realize that you have eaten a small amount and you're satisfied. You're in touch with your body and what it needs, and you stop when you're satisfied. You love the feeling of being inside your body and giving it what it needs. Count from 1 to 5 and let the scene play out, feeling relaxed and completely yourself. Noticing how wonderful and healthy you are . . . 1 . . . 2 . . . 3 . . . 4 . . . 5.

Now keep that wonderful feeling with you and let that scene fade away. Now, imagine yourself at some time in the future, a time when you are moving in healthy ways, letting your body be active. You might be walking, practicing yoga, taking the stairs instead of the elevator. Letting it come in clearly, and letting your unconscious mind show you the positive image it would like for you to experience. Feeling healthy and vibrant, full of life . . . Count from 1 to 5 and let the scene play out, feeling completely yourself and very satisfied. 1 . . . 2 . . . 3 . . . 4 . . . 5. Good.

Now keeping that feeling of being in a healthy body that moves easily and exactly as you would like, let that scene fade away. Imagine yourself now as your ideal self. In a healthy body, making healthy choices for yourself, living life fully every day, in every way. Make it as real as you can. Experiencing it completely, inside and out . . . Count from 1 to 5 and let the scene play out, feeling completely yourself, very satisfied and very beautiful. 1 . . . 2 . . . 3 . . . 4 . . . 5. Wonderful. Now let that scene fade away.

Here are some suggestions to your unconscious mind: You will accept all of these suggestions naturally and completely.

Your Personalized Scripts

Insert your scripts here:

Your intention:

_____

_____

Your belief self-suggestions:

_____

_____

Your behavior self-suggestions:

_____

_____

Coming Up Script

Now see yourself in the future: you have achieved your goal, you have accepted all these new beliefs, and you have changed your behaviors as you desire. Take a moment to let that image of yourself come in clearly. (Long pause.)

In a moment, I will count up from 1 to 5, and when I reach the count of 5 you will be awake and alert, having accepted all my suggestions. You will find these suggestions agreeable and easy to accept, and have, in fact, already integrated them into your life. You will act on them easily and naturally. At the count of 5 you will awake feeling wonderful, and will love being in your body. You will remain relaxed, but alert, for as long as you would like. When it is time to sleep, you will sleep well and will awake refreshed.

So, beginning to come up, counting . . . 1 . . . 2 . . . wiggling fingers and toes, feeling is coming back into them now . . . 3 . . . big deep breath, over halfway there now . . . shrugging your shoulders and making larger movements with the body . . . 4 . . . getting ready . . . and . . . 5! . . . _eyes open_ . . . wide awake and alert, now, feeling wonderful, motivated, and full of life!

Using this personalized tape will produce far better results for you than any prerecorded self-hypnosis tape you could possibly buy. Why? Because the work you put into it will make it far more meaningful for you than a one-size-fits-all tape. The fact that it is your own voice talking to you will further solidify the concept of getting in touch with your inner essence, tapping into your spirit, and finding the inner strength necessary to create the life (and the body) you want.

And this, after all, is the essence of the work we are doing here together.

This is the spirit of Molly Fox's Yoga Weight Loss Program.

Chapter Fifteen
The Best Diet Plan in the World

Eureka!
(I have found it!)

—Archimedes, Greek mathematician and inventor

We're going to tell you about an exercise that unequivocally enables us to make the following statement: It is the single best technique we have ever found for losing weight, keeping it off, and gaining an unbelievable amount of personal power in the bargain.

Yes, you heard right.

It takes no more than 10 minutes a day—usually less. It costs nothing. There's no equipment. There is no special diet involved—in fact, you can do it with any diet you happen to be following, although we recommend you use it in conjunction with Molly Fox's Yoga Weight Loss Program. But it's perfectly compatible with Jonny Bowden's Shape Up, Atkins, the Zone, Weight Watchers, Carbohydrate Addict's Diet, Paleolithic, Portion Control, or, God help us, even the USDA Food Pyramid. It doesn't matter. It complements every one of them.

And it is so elegantly simple that when we tell you how to do it, the cynical voice inside you—the one that takes up residence within each and every one of us and never seems to leave—is virtually bound to scoff, "That's ridiculous. It's too easy. It can't possibly work."

Don't listen to that voice.

If you use this tool in the way that we're going to tell you to use it, and you use it consistently along with this program, we will virtually guarantee you that you will see miracles happen in your life. One of those miracles is that you will lose weight.

The second is that losing weight will ultimately seem to be insignificant compared to what else you will get out of this program.

Let us explain.

Both of us have been coaching people on how to get results in their lives for a long time, but you have to understand: We're fellow travelers on this weight loss road. It's no easier for us than it is for you, and we understand as well as anyone the desire for a magic program, an instant fix, a stop-the-presses breakthrough in the theory and practice of dieting and weight loss. (Let us save you some time: It doesn't exist.) Although most of the time we maintain our weight where it should be and we exercise regularly, it is frighteningly easy for both of us to put fat on, and it takes a lot of focus for us to keep it off.

After Jonny's first book (*Shape Up!*) came out, and right before the publication of the second (*Shape Up Workbook*), he gained some weight and was having a fiendishly difficult time losing it. And he was not having a hard time because he didn't know how or what to eat. Jonny can discuss the biochemistry of weight loss and weight gain with anyone, including the contribution of hormones, enzymes, food allergies, genetics, metabolism, and psychology. If it's information that's legitimately out there in the field of weight loss and body transformation, you can bet that Jonny knows about it.

We're telling you this for one simple reason: It didn't matter.

It wasn't information that was stopping Jonny from losing weight. And it isn't information that stops you, either.

Look, if information were all we needed to change a habit, there wouldn't be any smokers, would there? Does anyone honestly think there's a smoker alive out there who doesn't know that cigarettes cause cancer? Do we really think that somewhere, someone hasn't gotten that bulletin yet, and as soon as they find out they'll say, "Gosh, I didn't know that, let me go throw these cigarettes away pronto!"

Oh, please.

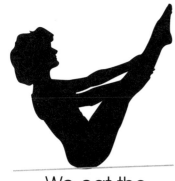

We eat the way we eat because it fills a function in our lives.

We eat the way we eat because it fills a function in our lives, a function that often goes unexamined. We eat unconsciously. We eat conveniently. We eat emotionally. And we eat in a way that actually expresses feelings and beliefs about ourselves, about who we are in the world, and about what we believe we can become (or what we don't believe we can ever become). And without looking at those issues, we will never really change the way we eat; we will never really lose weight and keep it off.

So the question for the day is this: What does how we eat, and what we eat, really say about what we believe ourselves to be?

These questions, though focused on food and eating habits, are very much true to the essence of a yoga practice. Throughout the book we have made references to connecting to a true and essential nature that is within each of us, and how, when you are really in touch with that, your daily choices in life tend to be life-affirming, joyous, and nurturing to your soul. The same is true with food. Unconsciousness is the devil's partner in weight gain. When you are more conscious of your essence and your purpose, it is much easier to move through life with freedom and ease. The weight (figuratively speaking) comes off your shoulders and the weight (literally speaking) comes off your body.

Let Jonny tell you in his own words how using the yoga-like tool discussed in this chapter altered the struggle he was having with his own weight.

So here I was, fresh from the success of my first books, which told people how to eat for weight management and optimal health, and yet I felt like my own weight was getting out of control. Although I was never more than 10 or 15 pounds from my ideal weight, this was a pretty big deal to me because, one, on my frame that weight really showed up, and two, because I was supposed to be the expert in this stuff. After all, people came to me to solve their weight management problems. I was nationally known as the "Weight-Loss Coach." And yet I couldn't seem to get my own weight problems under control!

One day, I woke up and got on the scale and then sat down at my desk and started to think about whether I really wanted to drop this last 10 pounds. (I did). Then I thought about what was getting in my way—what feelings, situations, places, things were cropping up that were keeping me from doing what I knew I needed to do.

And I spontaneously picked up a pen and paper, and began to write myself a letter.

I now call it "the Weight Loss Letter."

I'll tell you right now, it took some courage. I had to look at myself in the mirror, see stuff I didn't like on my body, admit it was there, and ask myself what I was going to do about it. I had to look at how long it's been there, and how long I'd been telling myself I'd take care of it "someday." It all poured out on the page. I let the pen take me wherever it needed to go. It was like written meditation. I just free-associated, thought about the situations I found myself in at night that caused me to eat in a way that I knew put that weight on (or at least kept me from losing it). I thought about what feelings I had in those situations, and how I felt after giving in to them. I filled exactly one page with this kind of written meditation, signed it "Love, Jonny" and put it away.

A remarkable thing happened.

That night, when I was in my familiar danger zone for overeating, I remembered what I had written in the letter. And I did not eat in quite the same way.

The next day, I weighed myself again. And started another letter.

I did this every day for 30 days. I lost 10 pounds.

In that month I discovered things about myself—connections between my eating behavior and ongoing issues in my life, my career, and my relationships—things that, believe it or not, I had never put together before. And I had accidentally discovered possibly the most powerful tool I had ever used in the field of weight loss.

How to Write Your "Weight Loss Letter"

So here's the drill.

Every morning, first thing in the morning, you're going to take a good look at your body. I suggest getting on the scale, naked, first thing in the morning before eating. Remember, this is an exercise in total honesty. Don't judge, just notice. Don't beat yourself up. Now sit down in a place where you will not be disturbed. Grab a fresh piece of paper and write yourself a letter about your weight and your body and your life.

Simple, right?

Give this technique 30 days in conjunction with this program. You will be astonished at the results it will produce.

Let's review.

Every single morning, for the next 30 days, you're going to weigh yourself, look at yourself, think for a moment, and then write yourself a one-page letter, for your eyes only. Include in it anything you want, but focus on your body, your eating habits, your trigger situations, what happened the day before, and especially what is likely to happen during the day that is about to begin. Visualize the unfolding day. What situations are you likely to find yourself in? What happens in those situations? What food will be available? How will you feel?

What will you do?

And, perhaps most important, how are your decisions and actions going to affect how you will feel tomorrow morning when you sit down to write again? How will the way you eat today make you feel tomorrow morning, when you get on the scale?

Always remember: Today is tomorrow's yesterday. When you examine yourself tomorrow morning and think back to how you ate last night and what you should have . . . could have . . . done instead, you will be talking about today. You can begin to eat mindfully and consciously right now and it will have an impact on the scale—if not tomorrow, then the next day or the day after.

By writing this letter and understanding this philosophy, you're going to begin to connect the action of everyday eating with the condition of being overweight. You're also going to begin to connect the action of your everyday eating with the unconscious statements you make to yourself about your body, your power, and your life.

You see, being overweight is a condition; eating something you don't really need is an action. We know they're logically connected—after all, when you eat too much, or eat the wrong stuff, you ultimately get fat. But because they're not connected in time, we don't always make the association at the moment the fork hits the mouth. When we take the action (overeating) we don't often think of the consequence (overweight) except in maybe some abstract sense. Why? Because they are so far apart in time. We don't have a lot of reinforcement for linking the action of eating to the condition of being overweight. We have no built-in system for bringing consciousness of the condition to the moment of choosing the action.

Until now.

Here are some examples of the way the Weight Loss Letter worked for some of our coaching clients.

Hal

Hal's downfall was nightly barhopping and munching on the free food at happy hour after work. Here's what he said in his letter:

I'm looking at the rolls of fat on my body and I'm not happy. Do I really want this weight to be there? Is how I feel about it right now in the cold light of morning worth the extra beer and peanuts with the guys at night? What do I really get out of that? Is it worth it? I can get these rolls of fat off and feel as great as I did in college. Is nightly beer and hot dogs worth giving up the feeling of power and strength I get from feeling my best?

Hal used that letter to start bringing consciousness of how he felt about his excess weight to the actions that were causing it. During that first week, he began to consciously think about what he had written in his morning letter while he was barhopping with the guys in the evening. He began to powerfully and emotionally connect those beer and peanut sessions with the feelings of defeat and powerlessness he'd feel in the morning when he'd look at his body, get on the scale, and see the results. He began to realize that he had the power to make a decision while in his "trigger situation" that would profoundly affect how he felt about his body the next morning.

Ashley

The frequent banquets and buffets that Ashley attended through her work in public relations were her undoing. Here's a sample from Ashley's letter to herself on a day when she knew she was going to face a particularly lavish banquet:

Will I let circumstances today dictate my personal power? They're going to put food in front of me. So what? Tomorrow when I write my morning letter I won't even remember how it tasted, but I'll remember the loss of my power. Theme for today: Circumstances aren't going to dictate to me my personal power.

Shannon

Shannon is a thirtysomething client who discovered that every time she got to a certain weight or reached a certain plateau she found some reason not to continue her program. Here's what she wrote in the second week:

I wonder if I'm not pushing as hard because I'm secretly "happy" at this weight, not willing to push the extra mile? Thinking "this is good enough." Theme for today: Let me find all the places where I stop myself in my life thinking "this is good enough."

Kim

Kim had an interesting situation going on. She was in a very unsatisfying relationship with what we came to call a "boyfriend of convenience." On some level, she just didn't believe she could "get" everything she really wanted in a man. Her "trigger situations" for unwanted eating centered around her roommates bringing home lots of TV munchies, junk food, and pizza. Here's an entry from one of her letters, a couple of weeks into the program:

Last night I ate a whole bunch of stuff because it was there. I think I do that in life as well. Go along because something's "there." Is that the kind of life I want? Do I want to have something—or be with someone—because he's there? Or because he's what I want? Am I willing to hold out for what I want or am I going to settle for taking what's there? And which kind of life do I want to have?

That night, Kim decided not to eat what was in the house just because her roommates brought it home. And shortly after, she broke up with the boyfriend and began setting out to find the kind of relationship she really wanted.

Here are a few other excerpts from clients' letters:

- Roberta wrote, "How in control of my life am I willing to be?" (As it turned out, very. Roberta lost 20 pounds over the course of 5 months and she feels—and looks—terrific.)
- Gerri, who ate compulsively when stressed, was able to anticipate the stressful situations and remember these words from one of her letters: "Today I choose to hold on to my personal power even—or especially—in the face of crisis." Gerri was able to completely revamp the way she responded to stressful situations with food, and to stay focused and conscious of her feelings instead, letting her make choices that supported her rather than sabotaging her life and weight loss goals.
- Anna traveled a lot and found airport eating a huge trigger. Air travel was very stressful to her, and she found that she would

"arm herself" with way more food than she needed. Here's an entry from one of her letters: "I need to watch out today for anxiety triggers as I'm very anxious about flying and about separating from my family. Today I will let myself experience that anxiety and not try to 'stifle it' with food I don't need. I will choose my food today based on what I need, not what I think I want. Today will be about gratitude—not greed."

▥ Sally wrote, "Today I am in the driver's seat of my life."

▥ Deidre, stuck at a plateau for a long time, wrote, "I wonder if I'm not pushing through because I'm secretly content to be this size. Maybe I'm thinking, 'this is good enough.'" Deidre used the weight loss letter to discover that she was really "cheating" a lot on her diet, and sabotaging herself with thoughts of "this is good enough" because at bottom, she didn't feel she could be bigger in life (and smaller in size!). Now she's both. Her self-imposed limitations were unconsciously keeping her from choosing what she needed to choose to expand her life and decrease her waistline!

The weight loss letter will help you to find out just where and how you put the brakes on being great. It will help you discover the statements you're really making about who you are in the world. It is guaranteed to make your eating behavior a lot more conscious, just at the time when you need that consciousness the most.

You will lose weight once and for all—or you will discover what gets in your way.

Or both.

And, like Sally, you will wind up feeling that you're "in the driver's seat of your life."

Conclusion
Putting It All Together—
the Yogic Lifestyle

I walked this way.
I walked that way.
And then I walked
my way.

—Chinese proverb

One of the central texts of yoga was written by Patanjali and is called the Yoga Sutras. The Sutras are more than 2,000 years old and contain the key to living a whole life based on integrity, health, and spiritual connection. They cover everything from an ethical code of conduct and a way of relating to the world to the development of a profound relationship to oneself and the Universal Presence.

This yogic path is made up of eight steps or "limbs" and it offers a system of transformation that can ultimately result in what is literally a "higher consciousness."

These eight steps, or eight limbs of yoga, are spoken about in Chapter 2 of Pantanjali's Yoga Sutras. They are:

1. Yamas: How we relate to others and the world.
2. Niyamas: How we relate to ourselves.
3. Asana: Our physical practice of poses.
4. Pranayama: Breathing practice.
5. Pratyahara: Withdrawing our senses inward.
6. Dharana: A single focus of directing our minds.
7. Dhyana: Developing a deeper relationship with a point of focus.
8. Samadi: Complete absorption with that point of focus.

The first two of these limbs basically establish the foundation for an ethical way of life. The third limb, asana, translates this into physical poses, much like those illustrated in this book and what you would do in a yoga class. And the fourth limb is concerned with breath. These first four limbs are considered "external practices" and can be passed on by instructor to student. They are considered preparations for the second four. These first four Sutras prepare our body, mind, and psyche—through discipline—for living in a way that honors our union with nature and the spiritual nature of our beings. They prepare us for meditation and deep absorption known in yoga as "essence." In this book, we have chosen to focus on the first five of the eight limbs, with special focus on the third, the asanas (physical poses). Part Three of this book focused on the fourth limb, pranayama (Breathing Practices), and the fifth limb, pratyahara (Meditations and Visualizations), which are meant to help you connect with your Essence.

The asanas—together with the eating program—are the most obvious tool you will be using to achieve your immediate physical goal of weight loss. We want you to remember, however, that while successful weight loss is the outcome of doing this program diligently, it is not the only result you will get. The big difference between most programs that concentrate only on weight, calories, and exercise, and the Yoga for Weight Loss Program is that the "traditional" slim-down programs do not take into account *the person losing the weight.* (Ayurvedic doctors are fond of making the following distinction between western medicine and eastern, and we think it applies here too. They say, *"In western medicine, the concern is with the disease. In eastern medicine, the concern is with the person having the disease."*) We believe this concern with the whole person is possibly the most important aspect of a program that changes the way you look physically (and feel emotionally) yet it is sorely neglected by most programs that concentrate only on diet and exercise.

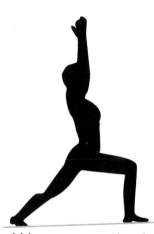

We are part of something much larger and more significant.

The yogic lifestyle begins with the thought that we are truly made up of the stuff of God. We are not merely what we do, where we live, who we are married to, and what we weigh, but rather, we are part of something much larger and more significant. This "something larger" is what we call our Essence. It is in all of us and it is in all things in the Universe. Our yoga practice ultimately brings us back home to this truth, so that we can live from our Essence more often.

It is always important to stay in touch with your "essence" when losing weight or making any major changes in your life, because we all too often allow ourselves to be seduced by the notion that we "are" what we look like, or we "are" just a number on a scale. Losing weight will undoubtedly change the way you see (and *feel about) yourself, and definitely the way others see you as well.* But it will not change who you are. It's important to stay in touch with that fact as the weight drops off and your appearance changes.

Many people have expressed an uncertainty to us about exactly what their "essence" is and how to get in touch with it. These questions are designed to help you do exactly that. Be thoughtful, but don't "think too much." Sometimes your first and most spontaneous association is the most revealing and truthful. You may find it useful to put these in your journal, and to return to them from time to time as more examples come to you.

Name some qualities that you feel are essential to who you are. *(Examples: love of animals, love of music, the feeling when I'm painting, etc.)*

_____

_____

_____

Name some experiences in your life where you feel you experience your essence. *(Examples: doing work that's meaningful, spending time with my grandchildren, making love)*

_____

_____

_____

As you see, yoga is about much more than just our bodies. We use our bodies to negotiate who we are in the world. Our bodies and our body language express a great deal about who we are, or who we think we are. Embracing and developing *who we really are* is the key to happiness.

As my teacher and mentor Michael Ray says, "There are two things you can count on, two things that are constant: Change and your enormous creative potential." Things are constantly changing—they're constantly in flux. This is just the nature of reality. To expect otherwise is to be in denial about the nature of life. Some changes are difficult, unexpected, and traumatic. Others are wonderful. But even amidst all this flux there is one thing that we can count on, and that is this deep well of creativity that we all have. It's this creativity that allows us to *deal* with change effectively. We often don't think we have this creativity or potential, but the truth is we do. It's from this deep well of personal resources that we come up with strategies to deal with change, or new creative ways to handle the kinds of things that come up in our lives.

For many of us, acknowledging that creative potential is difficult. Your inner critic will tell you that you're wrong—that you have no such creative source. It is here that the idea of faith really comes alive. It's precisely that deep well of creative consciousness that you need to have faith in. This creative energy is part of what we call our "essence." Believe in it, for it exists as surely as the book you are holding in your hand. Yoga is about *accessing* it.

Answer these three questions quickly, again without thinking too much. Just write down what comes up for you. You can write them right here, or in your journal.

What is it you really want to do?

_____

_____

How do you really want to live?

_____

_____

Who do you really want to be?

_____

_____

Pay attention to what came up for you when you answered these questions. Now ask yourself who was speaking—your inner critic? Or your Essence?

Looking at these things may end up making you more committed to where you are right now. You may find you have a new appreciation for the gifts you have been given. Or, you may choose to make a few changes. Or even some large and sweeping ones.

Remember, though, it is not just the changes that make the difference. It's getting in touch with what really matters to *you*. It is about much more than just "making changes," it is about being aware of who you are and *living your truth* that really counts. And that doesn't always mean change. It *might* mean making some hard choices, like staying put and working things out when you really want to run. Only you know what the real personal truth is, and that's the whole point.

Through your yoga practice you can create the *body* you want, and the *life* you want.

What would you like more of in your life?

_____

_____

What would you like less of?

_____

_____

What's missing in your life that, if you had it, would enhance the quality of your life?

_____

_____

Yoga Embodiments or "Life Practices"

We suggest spending a week or so with each of these "exercises," practicing the concept described. You will be amazed at the results.

Practice Love (Ahimsa)

To live with love means to do no harm and to see with your heart instead of with your head or your eyes. Focus this week on the love you have within you when everything else falls away including anger, fear, and resentment. Think of seeing the world this week from the eyes of the God within. Ask yourself the question: "What would God (as I understand him) want me to do?" See what comes up.

Write in your journal about what came up for you.

Practice Truth (Satya)

To live with truth means to live from your own personal truth; it means to dig deep inside, be courageous and look at the real truth in any given situation. Be aware of when you are fooling yourself or others. Notice where the truth comes up for you in your week.

Write in your journal about what came up for you.

Practice Happiness for Others (Asteya)

To live with happiness for others means to let go of jealousy for what someone else has. Living with happiness for others can also unlock the doors to you realizing just how much you have and finding what it is you truly want in life. Focus this week on the good you can do for others, on random acts of kindness, and on generosity. See what comes up for you.

Write in your journal about what came up for you.

Practice an Honoring of Your Sexuality (Brahmacarya)

Living with a deep respect of your sexuality honors the most natural of our Embodiments. We are, after all, human animals of a particular sex. Our sexuality is a very big part of what makes us what we are. It is keen to our mental health and our enjoyment of life. When it is undervalued or overvalued we become slaves to it and it becomes almost impossible to live from our Essence. When you do this exercise, live with a focus on honoring and accepting your own sexuality.

Write in your journal about what came up for you.

Practice a Deep Respect for the Simplicity of What Really Matters (Aparigraha)

To live with Respect for Simplicity steers us away from hoarding things. It can release us from the compulsion to buy more and more things that we think will make us free or happy. Accumulating more and more things—most of which we don't really need—simply encourages us to put our faith into things we can *buy* as opposed to putting our faith in who we really *are*: our Essence. Leading a simpler life, concentrating on the essential, the things that really matter to you—even if it's just for the week or so that you do this exercise—encourages you to be truly grateful for the presence of everything and everyone that you have.

Write in your journal about what came up for you.

Think of the feeling you get when your house or car is a mess. That mess—that "incomplete work"—takes up psychic space. Just consider how much better you feel when everything is spotless and clean. There is a sense of lightness that comes with order, with physical cleanliness, with the cleanliness of your home and the orderliness of your routine. All of that helps to reveal your Essence. For this exercise, live with that focus and see what comes up.

Write in your journal about what came up for you.

Practice an Acceptance of What Is (Samtosa)

Most of our unhappiness is rooted in our expectations that things ought to be different from the way they are. A lot of misery can be traced to our "should have beens" and "ought to bes". (Jonny once wrote of the "Bowden Equation: Unhappiness equals the distance between Reality and Expectation.") But the more we think something "ought" to be different from the way it is, the more we resist it. And "what you resist persists." From acceptance of what is—including, by the way, your weight—you can make the space to begin to move forward. Focus this week on letting things be the way that they are and the way they are not. See what comes up for you.

Write in your journal about what came up for you.

Most of us surrender our power on a daily basis. But that inner power is part of your Essence. It's your ability to get done what you want done. It's your own inner power and strength that you are practicing when you keep your word—when you *say* you are going to do something and then you actually *do* it. Live this week with an awareness of how powerful you really are. See what comes up.

Write in your journal about what came up for you.

That is what the yogic lifestyle is really about.

We hope that the tone and feel of the book expresses how profoundly we feel that yoga is much more than just poses or physical movement, just as *you* are much more than just your body. It is this sense of wholeness and integration that fundamentally separates yoga from simple exercise or weight loss programs. Those programs focus only on toning the body and changing a number on the scale.

As we've shown, yoga is truly a great way to lose weight.

Even more important, it is a way to live your entire life.